Evidence-Based Practice in Primary Care

Edited by

Leone Ridsdale MSc PhD FRCGP FRCPC

Reader in General Practice, Department of General Practice, UMDS Guy's and St Thomas' Hospitals, London

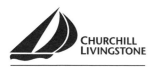

CHURCHILL
LIVINGSTONE

EDINBURGH LONDON NEW YORK PHILADELPHIA SYDNEY TORONTO 1998

CHURCHILL LIVINGSTONE
A Division of Harcourt Brace and Company Limited

© Churchill Livingstone, a division of Harcourt Brace
and Company Limited 1998

D is a registered trade mark of Harcourt Brace and
Company Limited

First Edition 1998

ISBN 0443 05889 X

British Library of Cataloguing in Publication Data
A catalogue record for this book is available from the
British Library.

Library of Congress Cataloging in Publication Data
A catalog record for this book is available from the
Library of Congress.

Medical knowledge is constantly changing.
As new information becomes available,
changes in treatment, procedures,
equipment and the use of drugs become
necessary. The authors and the publisher
have, as far as it is possible, taken care to
ensure that the information given in this
text is accurate and up to date. However,
readers are strongly advised to confirm that
the information, especially with regard to
drug usage, complies with current
legislation and standards of practice.

The
publisher's
policy is to use
**paper manufactured
from sustainable forests**

Printed by Bell & Bain Ltd, Glasgow

Contents

Contributors

Richard Baker, MD, FRCGP
Director of Eli Lilly National Clinical Audit
Centre, Department of General Practice and
Primary Health Care, Leicester General
Hospital

Jonathan Deeks, BSc, MSc
Medical Statistician at the Centre for
Statistics in Medicine, Institute of Health
Sciences, Oxford

Gene Feder, MD, FRCGP
Senior Lecturer at the Department of
General Practice and Primary Care, St.
Bartholomew's and the Royal London
School of Medicine and Dentistry at Queen
Mary and Westfield College

Chris Griffiths, MA, DPhil, MRCP, MRCGP
Senior Lecturer at the Department of
General Practice and Primary Care, St.
Bartholomew's and the Royal London
School of Medicine and Dentistry at Queen
Mary and Westfield College

Anthony Harnden, MRCP, MRCGP, DCH
Principal in General Practice, Morland
House Surgery, Wheatley, Oxfordshire

Peter Havelock, MBBS, FRCGP
Associate Adviser at Oxford University
Deanery and also a General Practitioner in
Buckinghamshire

Mayur Lakhani, MRCP, MRCGP
General Practitioner and Lecturer at Eli
Lilly National Clinical Audit Centre,
Department of General Practice and
Primary Health Care, Leicester General
Hospital

Tim Lancaster, MB, BS, MSc, MRCGP
General Practitioner at the Jericho Health
Centre in Oxford

Heather Lodge, BLib, ALA, MSc
Librarian in Public Health Medicine,
UMDS Guy's and St. Thomas' Hospitals,
London

Myfanwy Morgan, BA, MA, PhD
Reader in Sociology of Health, Department
of Public Health Medicine, UMDS Guy's
and St. Thomas' Hospitals, London

Irwin Nazareth MBBS, DRCOG, MRCGP, PhD
Senior Lecturer at the Department of
Primary Health Care and Population
Sciences based at the Royal Free Hospital
School of Medicine and at University
College London Medical School at the
Whittington Hospital

Leone Ridsdale, MSc, PhD, FRCGP, FRCPC
Reader in General Practice at the
Department of General Practice, UMDS
Guy's and St Thomas' Hospitals, London

Acknowledgements

In contrast to writing a book on one's own, editing a book is a more social process, and I have enjoyed this collaboration. I am particularly grateful to David Sackett, who suggested I contact Peter Richardson at Churchill Livingstone. Their support and encouragement got me started. The first evidence-based medicine workshop in Oxford and subsequent ones in London introduced me to like-minded GPs and specialists, and made me think of how these evolving skills might contribute to our understanding of different aspects of primary care. I am grateful to my collaborators for carrying this forward in their own areas of expertise.

My publisher suggested that at the end of some chapters it would help to reprint papers which provided important evidence to answer a question, so readers would have ready access to them. The *British Medical Journal*, Blackwell Science, *Journal of the American Medical Association* and the *British Journal of General Practice* all gave permission for papers to be reprinted, and the editors and publishers of *Evidence-based Medicine* gave permission for their glossary of terms to be reprinted at the end of the book.

Jonathan Deeks (Chapter 9) is grateful to Julie Parkes for reviewing the chapter and providing the case scenario. Permission for publication of the output from the COCHRANE LIBRARY has been given by Update Software.

Many people have read chapters and provided feedback for me, including Peter Cantillon, Lea Cramsie, Eric Saunders and Nigel Smeeton. Graham Dunn, David Sackett and Sharon Strauss provided feedback on the whole book. I am immensely grateful to all these people. Heather Lodge, as well as helping me in my searches, collaborated, and checked the references — thank you. Sarah Wilkinson helped me administratively in bringing the whole book together. Some quirks, biases and errors will remain all my own. Thanks finally to my family, au pairs and friends for support and forebearance throughout.

Preface

My wish to produce this book started as I reflected on what the book (Ridsdale 1995) I published with Saunders had left out. I had gradually introduced the skills involved in critical reading over the course of the book, with a section on critical reading and the philosophy of knowledge at the end. As soon as the book was published, friends and colleagues wrote to say that I stopped writing the book just when it was beginning to become more interesting, and they would like to see the last few chapters developed more. David Sackett's move to Oxford and the launching of courses on evidence-based medicine provided a stimulus for people who were explicitly interested in developing strategies for lifelong learning to talk together. Meeting fellow enthusiasts had a tonic effect on me. It has been challenging to get my mind around new aids to practice, like number needed to treat (Chatellier et al 1996). It has also renewed my interest in clinical medicine. Medicine is by no means the only ingredient of primary care, but it is easy to lose touch with it in the context of British general practice.

Kuhn (1970) made it clear that no paradigm is completely new; but putting established ideas together in a different way can lead to new ways of seeing things. The combination of ideas and methods included in evidence-based health care may lead to improved solutions to a perennial problem of how to continue learning-in-practice. This book is part of the process of bringing together emerging strategies for continuing learning, with primary care.

Since my first book was published I have intermittently been asked to give a lecture on an evidence-based approach to general practitioners and doctors on day-release or MRCGP revision courses. These invitations have made me concerned that learners could get the message that the knowledge, skills and attitudes embodied in this approach can be imbibed passively and / or at one sitting. On this account I have refused some invitations, or tried to negotiate for more time and preparation for learners, so that we can take a workshop approach. I hope this book may fill this sort of learning need, acting as a 'companion-guide', with readers using it on their own or to prepare for learning in a group context.

In preparing this book I have asked friends and colleagues who have contrasting interests and expertise to describe how to answer different types of question. These questions must be ones that they think are interesting, and they must be core problems in general practice. They are intended to exemplify the diverse approaches that are appropriate to answering questions in primary care. The questions we came up with are:

- What are parents' worries about acute illness in a child?
- How can we reduce diagnostic uncertainty when a patient presents with back pain?
- What is the long-term outcome for those who attend with psychological problems?
- How can the practice find and apply a strategy which is likely to be effective in reducing prescribing for sleeping pills?
- How can a practice find and apply valid guidelines for managing acute asthma?
- How might practitioners audit the quality of their diabetes care?
- Are antibiotics beneficial for children with otitis media?

Each contributor has described the knowledge and skills that are needed to find a useful answer to the question posed. The process involves defining (or teasing out) what the problem consists of, and searching for, appraising and applying evidence in relation to a particular issue in practice. Whilst the emphasis is on the process, I hope that readers will find some of the evidence uncovered interesting in itself.

I have not attempted to standardize the work of contributors, each of whom has his or her own style and identities. Apart from the first chapter, each chapter stands on its own, and chapters can be dipped into or read in any order. General practitioners are used to shifting their mental framework for each consultation, and in this context it seemed more natural for each contributor's chapter to be in his or her 'individual voice'.

Parents are inclined to tell their children to do what they say, and not what they do. This is perhaps because they know that the reverse is more common. Learners likewise model themselves on their mentors. Peter Havelock has stressed this in the final chapter on teaching and learning evidence-based practice. Those of us in primary care who want to facilitate learning need to be seen to be learning too. Setting up and sustaining this learning context is a challenge, especially whilst continuing to provide care that is both accessible and responsive to patients. The traditional medicine paradigm never required general practitioners to pose as experts, so we can — and many do — continue to learn with attitude. I hope that by doing this we can change both ourselves and the profession in useful ways; following in this spirit I invite readers to go on writing to tell me what has been left out.

References

Chatellier G, Zapletal E, Lemaitre D, Menard J, Degoulet P 1996 The number needed to treat: a clinically useful nomogram in its proper context. British Medical Journal 312: 426–429

Kuhn T S 1970 The structure of scientific revolutions. University of Chicago Press, Chicago

Ridsdale L 1995 Evidence-based general practice: a critical reader. W B Saunders, London

CHAPTER 1

Introduction

Leone Ridsdale

In primary care clinical observation, based on the history and examination, represents primary evidence. The clinical experience of the practitioner, both of this particular patient and of other patients, is also important evidence in the decision-making process. Practitioners use many different sources of information. For example, many computer packages which I and other general practitioners use only need the first few letters of a drug to be typed before they supply a list of the drugs which begin in this way, along with the usual dose of the drug selected. This stored information reduced the need for me to have it memorized, but when I work out of hours for our cooperative with no computer, I must either remember or look up the spelling and the dose of some drugs in the *British National Formulary*.

For some of the time in a busy practice I work almost unquestioningly in an 'automatic pilot' mode. At these times my overriding concern may be to catch up if I am running late, and not keep other people waiting too long. There is evidence that doctors ask fewer questions when they are busy (Ely et al 1992). At other times I recognize the limits of my knowledge and ask questions, especially if I know I can get the answer quite easily. For example, when patients ask about the vaccinations they need for a holiday, I immediately refer them to the practice nurse, who has all the necessary information on an up-to-date wall chart. If I am uncertain about some other aspect of medical management I may telephone someone else to get a second opinion. I am more comfortable about doing this if I know the person and find him or her approachable, but there are limitations to this method. As a trainee, I once asked an ear, nose and throat surgeon for information about the effectiveness of decongestants for children with glue ear. His answer took the form of another question. Would he use decongestants if they were not beneficial? This response troubled me as it discouraged me from questioning, and encouraged a view that he, because he was a senior doctor, was automatically doing things that were beneficent and/or right.

The move to evidence-based practice occurs in this continuous learning context. Sometimes I do not know when I am reaching the limits of my personal knowledge, or when there is actually insufficient evidence to answer a question. Having strategies and skills to explore this area of uncertainty is the nub of evidence-based practice.

The process of continuing learning

1. Questioning comes first. For me, having 'official' learners, like students and registrars, helps raise more questions. I then only need to acknowledge that I do not have the answer. This is not necessarily easy; it takes some confidence to disclose ignorance and uncertainty, and learners often want quick answers too. Once a question is posed it generally needs to be sharpened up before searching for information, or asking a librarian to do so. This process is described further in the next chapter.

2. I have already described some of my searching strategies. Some sources are close at hand: in the clinical notes, in my memory and clinical experience, in taking a good history and in examining the patient. Yet there are all sorts of external sources to tap if I have the time and motivation. Searching is the normal practice of librarians, and I have learned a lot from them, both about general practice and about the process of refining questions and searching. Heather Lodge has described this process in the next chapter.

3. Once we get hold of the papers we then need to appraise whether the evidence is reliable and valid, by using questions in relation to criteria which are designed to test the strength and weaknesses of the research. The tools and skills to appraise papers are evolving. Sackett et al (1997) have described how to appraise papers on clinical topics. This present book builds on their framework to describe critical appraisal in the context of primary care.

4. Next we need to decide the extent to which external evidence can help when it is applied to a patient or a policy in general practice.

5. Schön (1983) has introduced the idea of practitioners reflecting whilst practising. The process of reflecting on

learning-in-action needs to be visualized and mapped out by and for general practitioners. We need to reflect on whether our process of learning-for-practice is efficient and effective, and how it can be improved on in the future. Peter Havelock has described a multifaceted approach to this in Chapter 10.

What evidence is relevant?

What kind of evidence can we find in this way? For example, general practitioners and their patients often need to know whether antibiotics are more beneficial than doing nothing for otitis media. A randomized controlled trial (Burke et al 1991) and a systematic review of randomized trials (Rosenfeld et al 1994) will help meet this need for information. Appraising systematic reviews is not easy, and Jonathan Deeks has described an approach to doing this in Chapter 9. On the basis of Rosenfeld et al's evidence I used to tell the mother of a child with earache that I would need to treat seven children with a similar problem for one child to benefit in terms of an earlier recovery. This did not necessarily lead to a uniform response from the patient's point of view. Some parents said they would rather not have antibiotics for their child because the benefits do not seem to outweigh the potential risks, whilst other parents chose to have antibiotics, saying that it may be beneficial if their child is the one in seven. In 1997 a new systematic review changed my view of the likelihood of benefit, and this is included in Chapter 9.

Those who have championed evidence-based medicine emphasize randomized control trials as being the gold standard for judging the benefits and risks of a treatment; but in general practice there are many topics which are more similar to behavioural science, for which cross-sectional surveys and qualitative methods provide more appropriate evidence. For example, British general practitioners are responsible for a lot of screening and surveillance activity for their practice population. In this context they need to know the characteristics of those patients who come and those who do not come, for example for cervical screening. Here evidence from surveys like that of Coulter and Baldwin (1987) will help. For those who do not attend for cervical screening, members of the primary care team need to know why, and evidence from in-depth interviews with patients may help us understand their views (Orbell et al 1995). Guidelines on how to appraise evidence derived using qualitative methods are provided in Chapter 3. With this kind of evidence, practitioners may try different ways to make the service more acceptable to those who come and those who have not come, and understand and possibly respect the reasons for non-attendance.

Often the problems which patients bring in primary care have no easy answer, particularly psychological problems. The practitioner and the patient may still want to know what is likely to happen in the future. Guidelines to evaluating papers on prognosis are described in Chapter 5. Practitioners in the National Health Service are also required to participate in audit, and for many reasons the process has often not seemed particularly worthwhile. Part of our scepticism is associated with the process being imposed, involving more work and potentially providing a stick to beat our own backs. Part of the negative response, however, may be associated with confusion about how to evaluate an audit to see if it is worthwhile. Criteria with which to design and evaluate an audit are described in Chapter 8 in the context a doctor's wish to improve the quality of his diabetes care. So the evidence which informs general practice is as broad-ranging as the work itself.

The need for theory (as well as evidence)

General practice departments frequently started life in departments of epidemiology and public health medicine. In this context GP researchers learned hypothesis-testing methods which are related to Popper's notion of generating explanatory theories, and then trying to falsify them (Popper 1968); but his approach emphasized the importance of theory, as well as the importance of theory-testing. Some epidemiologists play down theory when they appraise evidence, making passing reference to other variables as 'confounders' in the analysis of data. If we want to make sense of or solve a problem in general practice, however, measurement is not sufficient on its own. We need to use our intuition to create imaginative theories, which are conjectures about what is going on (Medawar 1969). We can then place models and measurement in juxtaposition, using each to interrogate and improve on the other. This imaginative process of model-building can be done by anyone, from medical student onwards, and newcomers to the field are often better able to provide fresh perspectives (Kuhn 1970).

What are the barriers to GPs doing evidence-based practice?

I recently challenged a group of GPs who were studying for an MSc to present reasons for not doing evidence-based general practice. They were most obliging and came up with a lot of arguments. Firstly, they argued that they had worked hard to pass undergraduate examinations and most of them had passed the membership examination of the Royal College of General Practitioners too. They were comparatively experienced practitioners now and their patients believed in them. 'If it ain't broken', they said 'there's no need to mend it.' This was an argument for maintaining the status quo. Yet they also saw limits to this closed approach. Patients challenged them with questions for which they often did not have answers, and often their patients had searched for information about new tests and treatments, which they as doctors did not know much about.

They pointed out that as full-time GPs many of them were doing nine surgeries a week and one session on call, as well as spending a lot of time on policy-making and administration. They already worked, or were on call, for about twice the hours that constituted a normal working week. Responding to repeated cycles of government-led change has been disorientating, and they felt as if they were suffering from jet-lag. They feared that anything else new might lead them to burnout. Lack of time does pose a problem for GPs who are trying to keep up to date, especially as the field in which they need to keep up to date is much broader than it is for other medical practitioners.

The doctors also pointed out that they felt they were being exposed to an epidemic of 'evidence-based' guidelines. Often these were produced by specialists, who seemed unaware of the different prevalence of disease, and different predictive values of tests when doctors were working in the community. These self-selected groups of 'experts' often had allowed only a token input from GPs, and so their guidelines were unlikely to be useful for guiding decision-making in family practice. In this context these guidelines might restrict GPs' freedom to prescribe for and manage their patients appropriately. There are guidelines that deserve to be put in the bin, and others which deserve consideration. How to decide on their merits is described in Chapter 7 in the context of providing care for a man with asthma.

Implicit in the evidence-based approach is an acknowledgement that what was learned at medical school or subsequently may no longer be best practice. Evidence for new diagnostic tests and approaches to management does periodically change, and this will not automatically be known to doctors working at the coal-face. The challenge to practitioners to apply the best available evidence does generate performance anxiety (Katz 1984, Berkson 1993). This was a criticism levelled by medical graduates at McMaster University of the self-directed, continuous-learning approach (Ferrier & Woodward 1982). 64% of women graduates commented on the anxiety level that this approach created. This performance anxiety is not necessarily alleviated by 'defenders of the faith', who purport to show that most interventions are based on evidence (Gill et al 1996). Practitioners do not automatically have the skills to search out and appraise the information that is presented in journals. Guidelines to appraising a paper on diagnostic tests are described in Chapter 4 in the context of a patient with back pain. Guidelines on how to appraise an intervention to reduce prescribing of sleeping tablets are described in Chapter 6.

Groups that I have worked with have generated lots of other objections, irritations and phobic reactions (as well as advantages) to an evidence-based learning approach. In Britain evidence-based medicine (EBM) is sometimes seen by its opponents as coming from 'over there' (the Atlantic), with lots of nasty acronyms and arithmetic. Its opponents in other countries may read about Archie Cochrane and the Cochrane Centre in Oxford, and think EBM comes from over here! Conversely, some of those who think EBM is worthwhile compete to own, rather than disown, its parentage. Some try to steal the moral high ground, implying that other doctors are practising without the benefit of evidence. This is rather like the 'holistic' doctors, who seemed to imply that the rest of us were not integrating the psychosocial components into our practice. It is too early to write a social history and trace the developments of the different components of an evidence-based learning approach. Certainly evidence-based practice may scare those who are computer-phobic or technophobic; but British GPs are more likely to be experienced computer users than their hospital-based counterparts, and have traditionally fostered a problem-based, adult learning approach. Lack of access to databases, which used to be a barrier for family physicians, is also rapidly being reduced by advances in technology. Many practices have already obtained and are storing their own information sources, like 'Best Practice' on CD-ROM.

Evidence-based practice is no panacea. Many of these concerns, like a lack of time, are real and justified. The aim of this book is to reduce some barriers by introducing readers to the knowledge and skills which are the tool kit for evidence-based practice. Like a manual for learning to play tennis or ski, it will require practice. Some barriers, like overwork, will remain. These policy issues will require more than a book to iron out. Rapid dissemination of research findings with responsive up-to-date practice has been supported by policy makers in principle, but it will be a concept which is not fully realized in general practice if there is insufficient political will or resources allocated to it.

General practice is comparatively untilled from the point of view of research, which means that some searches yield little, or yield only answers from hospitalized patients which may not be applicable in general practice. This can be frustrating, but it can be reassuring to find that our knowledge limits in a particular area are also limits to scientific knowledge. A gap between relevant questions and answers is exciting and challenging to researchers. The scientific study of general practice is developing at a time when social scientists are also developing their techniques; so economists, sociologists, psychologists and others are refining methodologies and producing evidence that will help answer questions which are relevant to us in future.

References

Berkson L 1993 Problem-based learning: have the expectations been met? Academic Medicine 68: 79–88

Burke P, Bain J, Robinson D, Dunleavey J 1991 Acute red ear in children: controlled trial of non-antibiotic treatment in general practice. British Medical Journal 303: 558–562

Coulter A, Baldwin A 1987 Surveys of population coverage in cervical cancer screening in the Oxford region. Journal of the Royal College of General Practitioners 37: 441–443

Ely J W, Burch R J, Vinson D C 1992 The information needs of family physicians: case-specific clinical questions. Journal of Family Practice 35: 265–269

Ferrier B M, Woodward C A 1982 Career choices, work patterns and perceptions of undergraduate education of McMaster medical graduates: comparison between men and women. Canadian Medical Association Journal 126: 1411–1414

Gill P, Dowell A C, Neal R D, Smith N, Heywood P, Wilson A E 1996 Evidence-based general practice: a retrospective study of interventions in one training practice. British Medical Journal 312: 819–821

Katz J 1984 Why doctors don't disclose uncertainty. Hastings Centre Report 14: 35–44

Kuhn T S 1970 The structure of scientific revolutions. University of Chicago Press, Chicago

Medawar P B 1969 Induction and intuition in scientific thought. Methuen, London

Orbell S, Crombie I, Robertson A, Johnston G, Kenicer M 1995 Assessing the effectiveness of a screening campaign: who is missed by 80% cervical screening coverage? Journal of the Royal Society of Medicine 88: 389–398

Popper K R 1968 The logic of scientific discovery. Hutchinson, London

Rosenfeld R M, Vertrees J E, Carr J, Cipolle R J, Uden D L, Giebink G S, Canafax D M 1994 Clinical efficacy of antimicrobial drugs for acute otitis media: meta-analysis of 5400 children from 33 randomized trials. Journal of Pediatrics 124: 355–367

Sackett D L, Richardson W S, Rosenberg W, Haynes R B 1997 Evidence-based medicine: how to practise and teach EBM. Churchill Livingstone, London

Schön D 1983 The reflective practitioner: how professionals think in action. New York, Basic Books

Additional reading

Dunn G, Everitt B S 1995 Clinical biostatistics: an introduction to evidence-based medicine. Edward Arnold, London

Sackett D L, Haynes R B, Guyatt G H, Tugwell P 1991 Clinical epidemiology: a basic science for clinical medicine. Little Brown, Boston

CHAPTER 2

How to ask questions and search for the literature

Heather Lodge and Leone Ridsdale

Clinical problem 1

A nurse in LR's practice asked if there was evidence for the effectiveness of nurse-run clinics for asthma. She had been running the clinic for several years, and had decided to evaluate it for her nurse practitioners' course. Ideally, the practice might have asked this question and done a search prior to starting the clinic! The nurse's question, however, provided the stimulus for her to visit HL, our local librarian, with a view to refining the question and learning how to search. HL's explanation of her approach to this important problem is described later in this chapter.

Clinical problem 2

LR worked for the cooperative on Saturday night doing the base surgery. Her registrar sat in and discussed the problems we saw. Most of the patients were worried mums bringing their children with infections. For those children with earaches we discussed whether antibiotic therapy made any difference. The registrar was keen to practise a search on MEDLINE, which he had access to through the *British Medical Journal* (*BMJ*) library service. We decided that we would define the question in advance. The clinical problem was otitis media. Parents came because they wanted antibiotics, so this was the intervention. The outcome which they and we ourselves might be interested in would probably be a reduction in the duration of symptoms in the short run. This outcome might be construed as a 'benefit', or more accurately harm avoided. LR's trainee decided that he was interested in results from a randomized controlled trial.

Introduction

This chapter aims to demonstrate that you do not need to be an information expert in order to find valuable information.

Clinical problem 3

Mr B came to see another nurse in our practice for a diabetes check-up. The patient had not been checking his blood levels, and the blood test the nurse had done showed his blood glucose was very high. She asked what was known about the beliefs of people like Mr B. The topic of interest was diabetes, and the context was general practice. We were not particularly interested in an intervention, but we were interested in health beliefs and in understanding health behaviour. We thought that MEDLINE might be less suitable for a search on this topic. As we were going to the local hospital for a lecture, we decided to ask our librarian for a good database to search on.

Clinical problem 4

A man came in asking LR for a sick note for back pain. He has four young children, and drove a taxi until last year. He has had back surgery on two occasions. It made LR wonder what patients think of their back pain management in general practice. She was busy that day and thought she would limit her search to a hand search of recent *BMJs* and the *British Journal of General Practice (BJGP)* which she keeps at home. The elements of this search were fairly straightforward. The problem or subject area was back pain. The context was general practice, and the object of the exercise was that she should learn more about patients' views. A quick trawl through the College journal was rewarding. She found a paper titled 'Patients' views of low back pain and its management in general practice' by Skelton and colleagues in the *BJGP* of March 1996.

Clinical problem 5

Mrs D came to the practice because she was feeling dizzy. She was so unwell that she had to lie down in the waiting room. When she came in to see LR she said she was upset because the specialist had put her on 'rat poison' for her atrial fibrillation. She asked if she could go back to using aspirin. LR's trainee was particularly good on therapeutics, so she asked him for his opinion. The problem here was atrial fibrillation. The intervention was warfarin versus aspirin. The benefit or harm avoided was probably stroke and death. LR's trainee was sure that warfarin was more beneficial than aspirin, but neither could be sure of the risk. Mrs D was clearly worried about the risk of haemorrhage or death, and we could not tell her precisely whether this outweighed the benefit. The trainee was keen to learn more about using the Cochrane database of systematic reviews. He volunteered to see HL about this and to report back to the patient and LR.

It should help you begin to think about how you can ask and answer questions prior to sitting at a computer. In all probability there is no such thing as a 'perfect search', and librarians do not hold a monopoly on being good searchers. All that is required is the ability to think around a subject, and scepticism about the infallibility of the computer. Most of the examples given in this chapter refer to MEDLINE because it is the most widely available database and the one with which general practitioners are likely to be the most familiar. For a selection of alternative databases, see Table 2.1.

Table 2.1 Summary of databases

Database name and producer	Scope	Availability
MEDLINE (National Library of Medicine, USA)	*Number of journals*: 3600 *Bias*: English language; strong American bias *Thesaurus*: Uses Medical Subject Headings (MeSH) *Subject coverage*: All specialties of medicine *Materials indexed*: Letters, editorials, research articles from 1966 onwards; 60% of references contain abstracts *Update*: Updated monthly but can be 3 or more months behind *Type of database*: Bibliographic	Free dial-up access to British Medical Association (BMA) members (cost of telephone call); Contact BMA for details and password; accessible via the Internet at the following sites: http://www.ncbi.nlm.nili.gov/PubMed *or* http://www.healthgate.com/HealthGate/MEDLINE/search.sbtml *or* http://www.medseape.com. Otherwise usually available in Postgraduate Medical Centres on CD-ROM
EMBASE (Elsevier Science Publishers, Netherlands)	*Number of journals*: 3500 journals *Bias*: European in focus *Thesaurus*: Uses own thesaurus *Subject coverage*: Strong on pharmaceutical and clinical medicine *Materials indexed*: Letters, editorials, research articles from 1974 or 1981 onwards (depending on method of access); overlap with MEDLINE estimated at between 25 and 40%; 75% of references have abstracts *Update*: Updated weekly and is about 4 weeks behind *Type of database*: Bibliographic	Accessible via the Bath Information and Data Services (BIDS) and available via most academic libraries; also accessible via the Internet at http://www.bids.ac.uk; one password required to access all BIDS databases; greater range of years available if a mediated search is done through a librarian via an online host
PSYCINFO (American Psychological Association)	*Number of journals*: 1300 *Bias*: English language material with North American bias *Thesaurus*: Uses own thesaurus but not as structured as MeSH or EMBASE *Subject coverage*: Psychology, psychiatry, sociology and linguistics: some overlap with SOCIAL SCIENCES CITATION INDEX. *Materials indexed*: Research articles, letters, editorials, books and chapters	Available on CD-ROM in academic medical libraries, associations such as British Medical Association (BMA), psychiatric hospital libraries and some postgraduate medical centres; worth tracking down if psychology/sociology is your particular interest

Table 2.1 *Cont'd*

Database name and producer	Scope	Availability
	letters, editorials, books and chapters in books from 1984 onwards, with about 75% being journal articles *Update*: Updated monthly *Type of database*: Bibliographic	
SCIENCE CITATION INDEX (Institute for Scientific Information, USA)	*Number of journals*: 4500 *Bias*: American *Thesaurus*: None; search using synonyms and keywords *Subject coverage*: Science and technology, life sciences, neuroscience, environmental science, statistics, public health; some overlap with MEDLINE and EMBASE *Materials indexed*: Research articles, letters, editorials, discussions, conference abstracts and book reviews from 1981 onwards; citation facility allows searching to identify articles quoting a specific study *Update*: Updated weekly and is 2 or 3 weeks behind *Type of database*: Bibliographic	Available via Bath Information and Data Services (BIDS) over the Internet or through academic medical libraries; BIDS Institute for Scientific Information (ISI) databases available only to academics; requires password
SOCIAL SCIENCES CITATION INDEX (Institute for Scientific Information, USA)	*Number of journals*: 1400 *Bias*: American *Thesaurus*: None; search using synonyms and keywords *Subject coverage*: Social sciences, anthropology, education, ethnic studies, industrial relations, psychology and sociology; some overlap with PSYCINFO and MEDLINE *Materials indexed*: Research articles, letters, editorials, discussions, conference abstracts and book reviews from 1981 onwards; citation facility allows searching to identify articles quoting a specific study *Update*: Updated weekly and is 2 or 3 weeks behind *Type of database*: Bibliographic	Available via Bath Information and Data Services (BIDS) over the Internet or through academic medical libraries; BIDS Institute for Scientific Information (ISI) databases available only to academics; requires password
UNCOVER (UnCover, USA)	*Number of journals*: 15 000 *Bias*: American *Thesaurus*: None; search by journal title or subject keywords *Subject coverage*: Multidisciplinary, from the end of 1988 onwards *Materials indexed*: Contents pages; copies of articles can also be ordered through UNCOVER and sent directly to you (giving you the cost in US dollars first!) *Update*: Very up to date *Type of database*: Bibliographic	Available via BIDS over the Internet or through academic medical libraries; requires password

Table 2.1 *Cont'd*

Database name and producer	Scope	Availability
COCHRANE LIBRARY (BMJ Publishing)	*Journals*: Does not scan journals; is a review database, bringing together articles from MEDLINE and EMBASE. Advantage is knowing that the articles listed are all recognized as controlled trials or systematic reviews *Bias*: None apparent *Thesaurus*: MeSH plus keywords *Subject coverage*: Clinical medicine reviews *Materials indexed*. A value-added database designed to provide evidence to support health care decisions; compiled by the Cochrane Collaboration and the UK National Health Service Centre for Reviews and Dissemination at the University of York; divided into four databases *Update*: Updated quarterly and is the source to consult for finding best evidence *Type of database*: Value-added	Increasing availability, including BMA, academic medical libraries and some postgraduate medical centre libraries. University of York's databases accessible via Internet at http://www.york.ac.uk/inst/crd/info.htm
DHSS DATA (Department of Health Library, UK)	*Number of journals*: 2000 *Bias*: British *Thesaurus*: Own *Subject coverage*: Health service and hospital administration, with particular emphasis on the UK; includes rarely indexed journals such as *Health Service Journal*; some overlap with MEDLINE on journal titles *Materials indexed*: Journal articles and other materials such as books and policy guidelines from 1983 onwards *Update*: Updated weekly but can be behind *Type of database*: Bibliographic	Not yet available on CD-ROM and therefore most frequently accessed through medical librarians using an online host; can be costly

Almost every request for information can be turned into a literature search using a three-stage process, known by the acronym PIE:

1. Plan the strategy.
2. Implement the search.
3. Evaluate the results.

Providing care is taken at the planning stage, and your request is reasonable, the PIE process should help you clarify the question. From there it should lead you to the appropriate source in which to look for an answer. Figure 2.1 illustrates

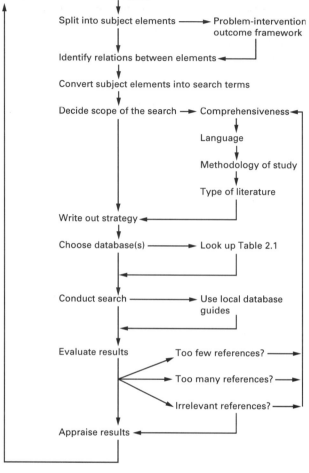

Fig. 2.1
Flow Chart illustrating the process of literature-searching.

the process of a literature search as a flow diagram. Each stage contains a number of steps to guide you through the process.

In order to illustrate the application of the principles to practice HL has used the first clinical problem and highlighted a sample search for information about the effectiveness of nurse-led asthma clinics throughout the chapter.

Splitting a query into subject elements focuses your thoughts; by doing so, the concept of asthma nurses in a hospital setting has been eliminated as being of no direct relevance in this case.

> A nurse in the practice is organizing a nurse-led
> asthma clinic but wants to be sure that it is worthwhile.
> This thought contains the following concepts:
> Asthma / Nurses / General practice / Effectiveness.

Stage 1: Planning the strategy

A search strategy is a logical series of statements that
translates a question into a meaningful search.

There are four steps in this stage:

a. Identify the subject elements of the question.
b. Define the relationship between the subject elements.
c. Convert the subject elements into search terms.
d. Decide on the scope of the search.

a. Identify the subject elements of the question

The first step in this strategy is to split a question into
separate subject elements. If the initial question proves
difficult to define or there are no obvious subject elements,
the Problem-Intervention-Outcome framework is a good
method to adopt. The above example could be shown thus:

> Problem: Asthma
> Intervention: General practice nurse
> Outcome: Effectiveness.

b. Define the relationship between the subject elements

The second step employs the use of tools that are
mathematical in origin. They are the means by which the
elements of a search are linked together in a logical way.
They are used in every search in any database. The three
tools, or operators, are: AND — OR — NOT.

AND

This operator requires each element to appear in the same
record. In Venn diagram terms, it is the overlap between two
or more sets. Figure 2.2 illustrates this. The shaded section in

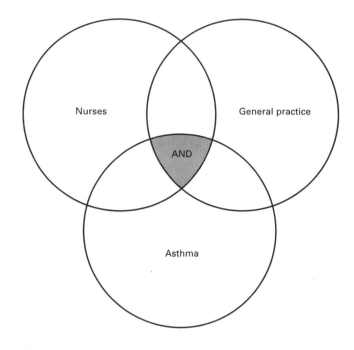

Fig. 2.2
Use of AND.

the middle represents the following relationship: Asthma AND General practice AND Nurses. The more elements that are connected using AND, the more specific the search will be.

OR

This operator requires either element to appear in a record. In Venn diagram terms, there is no overlap between any set. Figure 2.3 illustrates this, and represents the relationship: Asthma OR General practice OR Nurses. Any duplicates will be omitted; thus the result of this search might not be the sum of its individual elements. For instance, the search might retrieve 30 references on asthma, 30 on general practice and 30 on nurses. Using OR to combine each of the three elements might result in a total of 78 references. Twelve references, therefore, have two or more of our terms in them. The more elements that are connected using OR, the broader the search will be.

NOT

This operator requires one element but not another to

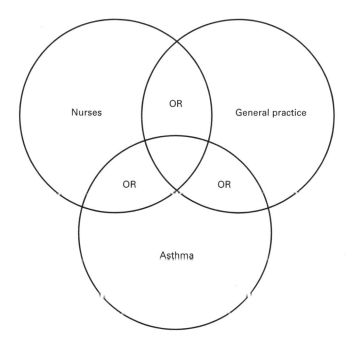

Fig. 2.3
Use of OR.

appear in a record. In Venn diagram terms, this is the set remaining after excluding another set. Figure 2.4 illustrates the effect of using NOT, and represents the relationship: Asthma NOT General practice. NOT is particularly useful for excluding a specific aspect of a subject. The example above would exclude a record which compared asthma in both the general practice setting and a hospital. NOT should be used with caution, as it can exclude comparative studies that could be relevant. For example, asthma NOT child will concentrate on adult asthma, omitting those records which discuss both adult and childhood asthma.

> The relationship between the elements in the search for a practice asthma nurse can now be determined. Using the operator AND, the search strategy is beginning to take shape thus: Asthma AND Nurses AND General practice AND Effectiveness

c. Convert the subject elements into search terms

The subject elements can now be translated into terms by

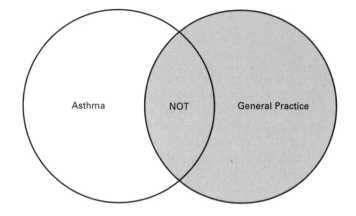

Fig. 2.4
Use of NOT.

which references can be retrieved. This step can be the most difficult to achieve and absolute accuracy is virtually impossible. There are two ways of searching and the most comprehensive search will make use of them both.

Free text or uncontrolled language

The first method of finding terms to express a subject comprehensively is to use free text or textword searches. This matches words with those that the authors might have used in the title, abstract or author keywords. The use of truncation, or abbreviating a word to its stem, is a good method of covering a lot of options. For example, use 'nurse$' to find 'nurse', 'nurses', 'nursed', 'nurse-led' etc. Free text is a very good approach if the subject is new or extremely specific – fundholding is a good instance of this and might appear as 'fundholder', 'fundholders' or 'fundholding'.

One disadvantage of this approach is that incorrect references are often retrieved; these are known as false drops. For example, a quick textword search in MEDLINE on fundholding brought up one or two references on student fundholding as well as many on general practice fundholding. This method also relies on the searcher having identified as many synonyms as possible to cover all eventualities, although if the author has not used the word the article has no chance of being retrieved.

Controlled language

Listing synonyms is a useful exercise; however, many databases use a controlled vocabulary and they index references accordingly. Clinicians, in contrast to librarians, start with a powerful advantage when it comes to literature searching because a number of the most accessible databases use a common vocabulary. The National Library of Medicine in the United States created a highly structured thesaurus to cover medical terminology for the purpose of indexing articles in MEDLINE. This is known as the Medical Subject Headings, or more familiarly as MeSH. Although increasingly sophisticated software, such as that marketed by Ovid Technologies, attempts to overcome the need to have an expert knowledge of MeSH, some awareness of its structure is still very helpful. Indexers are instructed to be as specific as possible in assigning terms to an article: for example, using 'osteoarthritis' rather than the broader term of 'arthritis'. The structure of the thesaurus allows the searcher either to concentrate on specific subjects or to bring individual elements together using the explosion facility. Both EMBASE and MEDLINE adopt this practice. A system of subheadings allows a precise aspect of a subject to be defined: for instance, the drug rather than diet treatment of arthritis would be indexed as arthritis/drug therapy. Lowe and Barnett (1994) wrote a comprehensive guide to understanding MeSH that is worth reading.

> In our sample search we might want to expand the specific diagnosis of asthma to include all respiratory tract diseases. The search would then use the explosion option to include all the diseases listed under 'respiratory tract diseases', of which asthma is one.

Apart from reducing the need to think of synonyms, a controlled language often allows the weighting of terms. During indexing, those terms that describe the most important aspects of an article are flagged, enabling attention to be focused on articles of direct relevance. This can be a useful method of controlling a search that retrieves hundreds of references. However, it should be remembered that weighting (also called majoring or focusing) a search assumes that both the searcher and the indexer agree on the elements that are of greatest importance in an article.

One of the disadvantages of a thesaurus is that the searcher has to rely on the indexers to apply headings consistently across the database, as well as having understood the article in the first place. Remember that indexers are most likely to be information professionals, who have only read the author's abstract and possibly the conclusions. If the abstract fails to describe the article adequately — omitting the methodology of a trial, for instance — the appropriate headings cannot be assigned.

A diversion on controlled language

At this point the subject of searching for randomized controlled trials may be of interest, as it has become the focus of much debate among both medical librarians and clinicians. The inadequacies of MEDLINE in identifying articles that have used this methodology have been described by Dickersin et al (1995), who carried out a search to test the accuracy with which trials could be retrieved from MEDLINE. They found that 'a MEDLINE search, even when conducted by a trained searcher, yielded only 51% of all known trials.' Measures are being taken to overcome this rather alarming figure but, as Dickersin et al point out, 'until editors require adequate description of study methodology in the title or abstract ... of every article published we cannot expect adequate indexing. Indexers can apply a study design term only if authors explicitly describe the design.'

The National Library of Medicine has begun to tackle the problem in response to the Cochrane Collaboration's concerns that trials are being 'lost'. A new indexing term of 'controlled clinical trial' was added to MeSH in 1995, being applied to studies that could not be described with certainty as randomized. MEDLINE's indexers are now more aware of the problem and are making efforts to describe the methodology. This is also being applied retrospectively as the UK Cochrane Centre identifies randomized trials that have not been indexed as such. This also applies to other database producers, such as Elsevier's EMBASE, which has also introduced the term 'randomized controlled trial' into its thesaurus.

The second clinical problem mentioned at the start of this chapter, whether antibiotics are valuable in treating otitis media, illustrates the difficulties of finding studies which are controlled trials. The search strategy for MEDLINE exploded 'otitis media/drug therapy' and 'antibiotics/therapeutic use'. This was then combined with the study methodology by exploding 'controlled trials' (to include randomized controlled trials) and using textwords such as 'controlled trial$', and 'random$ trial$', as well as using the term 'clinical trials' from the list of publication types. The results were restricted to those articles in English, with abstracts and about children. The following paper was retrieved: Burke P et al 1991 Acute red ear in children: controlled trial of non-antibiotic treatment in general practice. British Medical Journal 303:558–562.

To return to our example search, we can add another stage to the strategy by finding synonyms and MeSH vocabulary:

- Synonyms:
  — general practice, general practitioners
  — nurses, practice nurses, special nurses, asthma nurses
  — effectiveness, cost-effectiveness
- MeSH:
  — asthma = asthma
  — general practice = family practice. general practitioners = physicians, family
  — practice nurses = nurses, nurse practitioners, nursing staff
  — effectiveness = cost benefit analysis

The final strategy will include a combination of MeSH and synonyms to be searched as textwords.

---

d. Decide on the scope of the search

The final step to planning the search strategy is to decide what is wanted from the search. This will often determine the choice of database. (See Table 2.1 for a summary of a selection of databases.) Step 4 asks the following set of questions.

How exhaustive is the search going to be?

Most databases will have between 15 and 20 years' data available; MEDLINE is unique in dating back to 1966. Most of them will also allow a search to be limited to the last few years.

> Since general practice asthma clinics are a recent innovation, the search can be restricted to the last 5 years' literature.

What about articles in languages other than English?

Dickersin et al (1995) found that between 18 and 20% of relevant trials in MEDLINE were not in English. Some subjects have been more extensively studied in Europe.

> Since our practice is in Britain, articles in German, for instance, may not be of the first importance. However, if we find nothing of immediate relevance in English, something else could still be of value.

Is a particular methodology relevant?

Despite the failings of the databases, it is still valuable to know if anything published is going to be useful or whether something more specific is wanted.

> We might consider a qualitative study in order to help evaluate patient opinions about a nurse-led clinic, as well as a randomized controlled trial or other review.

What type of literature is relevant?

The type of literature required will determine where the search is carried out. EMBASE and MEDLINE are very good for clinical articles but for something more sociological the SOCIAL SCIENCES CITATION INDEX or PSYCINFO may be more appropriate (see Table 2.1). Health policy information and practice guidelines can be a different challenge altogether.

The third clinical question raised at the start of this chapter on patients' beliefs about diabetes is a good example of a search worth trying in PSYCINFO. Searching using the terms 'diabetes' and 'health attitudes' and restricting this to articles in English with abstracts retrieved, among others, we found the following reference: Murphy E and Kinmouth A L 1995 No symptoms, no problem? Patients' understandings on non-insulin dependent diabetes. Family Practice 12:184–192.

> Our sample search seems to be a clinical question but a venture into the sociological literature might yield some interesting studies.

End of stage 1: Conclusions

The initial search strategy can now be created by bringing together the decisions made at each of the four steps described above. These steps provide a starting point to begin searching but it is likely that some refinements will have to be made as the search progresses.

> The original idea has now been developed into the following quest for information: a randomized controlled trial and/or qualitative study that has been done in the last 5 years, preferably in Britain, on:
> Asthma
> AND
> Family practice OR Physicians, family
> AND
> Nurses OR Nurse practitioners OR Nursing staff OR Practice nurse
> AND
> Great Britain
> AND
> Cost benefit analysis OR Effectiveness.
> This uses a mixture of MeSH and textwords, since the concept of a practice nurse has no direct match in MeSH and effectiveness is not well covered.

The strategy creates a matrix, with synonyms forming the rows and the subject elements forming the columns. The operator OR is always used in rows. The operator AND is nearly always used in columns; the exception is in textword searches which are looking for a phrase rather than one word: practice AND nurses, for example.

If this strategy produces hundreds of references, the methodology can be added into the search. In theory this should just be 'randomized controlled trials' as a type of publication. Using MEDLINE under the Ovid software, this is added by choosing the option to limit a search and selecting from a list of limits including English language articles, specific age groups and publication types. In practice a combination of textwords such as 'random', 'controlled', 'clinical trial', and MeSH terms including 'randomized controlled trial', 'controlled clinical trial', 'double blind method', 'single blind method', 'evaluation studies', 'prospective studies' and 'comparative studies' are needed as well as the publication type.

Stage 2: Implement the search

It is now time to test out the strategy by searching a database for articles that include the subject terms. There are two steps to this stage, at the end of which a number of references should have been found to follow up.

a. Identify appropriate databases.
b. Conduct the search.

a. Identify appropriate databases

Table 2.1 is a brief guide to some of the major systems that are used regularly by medical librarians. Every librarian has a favourite and every librarian will say that the list omits more than it includes. The choice of database is growing wider every year but MEDLINE remains the most popular. It is also likely to be the most readily available database for general practitioners to access, particularly now that the National Library of Medicine has made MEDLINE freely available over the Internet. However, Lefebvre (1994) points out that 'only c.3700 of the c.15 000 biomedical journals received by the National Library of Medicine are indexed for MEDLINE.' Concentrating a search exclusively in MEDLINE, therefore, may provide an adequate answer to an enquiry but is unlikely to be a complete answer, as valuable references may have been indexed elsewhere.

You need to be aware of what exists and what might realistically be available to you. Limiting your search to a scan of journals readily available may be enough to find a perfectly adequate answer, as long as you are aware that this is not the ultimate literature review. As was demonstrated in Clinical problem 4, the question of what patients thought about their treatment of back pain in general practice was answered satisfactorily by scanning the contents pages of the *British Journal of General Practice*.

> For our example on asthma nurses, a selection of databases, beginning with MEDLINE and following through to EMBASE and SOCIAL SCIENCES CITATION INDEX, is the best option. If time and effort were unlimited it might also be worth requesting that a librarian search DHSS DATA for policy statements.

b. Conduct the search

The second step is to put the theory into practice by logging on to a database and typing in the terms. It would be neither feasible nor appropriate to attempt to describe the exact sequence of commands required by a system in order to achieve this step. This is best left to the many excellent guides that exist. If you are doing a search in a library, try using the guides produced by the librarian. They will be specific to the software and machines in that library. In addition, Bath Information and Data Services (BIDS) produce two useful introductions to the Institute for Scientific Information databases and EMBASE. Contact the BIDS team at Bath University or via their Internet address (see Table 2.1). Lee and Millman's (1996) *ABC of Medical Computing* includes a chapter on how to search MEDLINE via the BMA library and a mine of information on searching using the Internet. Robert Kiley's (1996) *Medical Information on the Internet* is also a very useful analysis of relevant sites.

Types of database

There is a gradual shift in the type of database available to searchers now that technology can provide much greater information storage capacities along with the ability to handle increasing volumes of data. A search may retrieve entire articles as well as a list of references.

Bibliographic databases

The most common type at present, these databases index the bibliographic reference. Each record comprises a number of fields, including the basic elements of the reference along with terms from MeSH or other thesaurus where used, the type of publication (e.g. letter, editorial etc.) and the language of the article. Thus a search will retrieve the author, title, source and abstract if there is one but not the entire article. Some CD-ROM systems will also provide a local location for journals.

Full-text databases

These databases store the complete text of a publication rather than just the references of articles within journals. Full-text databases are increasingly available and range from newspapers such as the *Guardian* to journals such as the *Lancet*. For the cost of a phone call the Internet provides access to an increasing range of information sources free of charge. Most journal publishers now post the contents pages of the latest issue on their web sites. The more interesting developments are those like the Doctor's Desk site, set up by St George's Hospital Medical School. Visit this site at http://drsdesk.sghms.ac.uk/ and you will find a wealth of valuable material, including links to full text evidence-based medicine sources such as Bandolier, Effectiveness Matters and ACPOnline. Ovid Technologies has now brought together the full text of 15 of the top medical journals, including the *BMJ* and *Lancet*, in one database called CORE BIOMEDICAL COLLECTION. In addition to searching the title and abstract, the rest of the article can also be searched. These databases mean that there is no delay between doing the search and reading the articles found as a result.

Value-added databases

Databases such as the COCHRANE LIBRARY are setting new trends in searching the medical literature by providing the searcher with some indication of the value of previously published research. The COCHRANE DATABASE OF

SYSTEMATIC REVIEWS is a full text database included as part of the COCHRANE LIBRARY. It comprises completed reviews of previous research and this material cannot be found in any other database. The DATABASE OF ABSTRACTS OF REVIEWS OF EFFECTIVENESS (DARE), compiled by the NHS Centre for Reviews and Dissemination at the University of York, is also part of the COCHRANE LIBRARY. Although this is not a full-text database it is value-added, as the reviewers at the Centre comment on how good the review is and assess the implications for practice.

The COCHRANE DATABASE OF SYSTEMATIC REVIEWS proved to be a valuable resource in answering the question on the use of warfarin versus aspirin. A search using the term 'atrial fibrillation' revealed the following review Koudstaal P 1996 Secondary prevention following stroke or transient ischemic attack in patients with nonrheumatic atrial fibrillation: antiplatelet therapy versus control. In: Warlow C, van Gijn S, Sandercock P Stroke module of Cochrane Database of Systematic Reviews, issue 2. Oxford, Update Software.

End of stage 2: conclusions

The search should have yielded some references to follow up.

If you try the example search on asthma nurses in general practice for yourself you should find the following useful references:

- Charlton I et al 1995 Asthma at the interface: bridging the gap between general practice and a district general hospital. Archives of Disease in Childhood 70: 313–318
- Charlton I et al 1992 An evaluation of a nurse-run asthma clinic in general practice using an attitudes and morbidity questionnaire. Family Practice 9: 154–160.

Stage 3: Evaluate the results

Stage 3 is concerned with evaluation. However much care is taken at the planning stage, further refinements are nearly always necessary to achieve a satisfactory result. Searching the literature in any discipline is about balancing precision or specificity against recall or sensitivity. The aim is to retrieve enough information to enable the decision-making process to take account of all relevant evidence. This has to be traded against finding either too much or too little evidence. Precision and recall used to be the subjects of lectures in a librarian's training. They are now the concern of every searcher.

- Precision or specificity is defined as the proportion of relevant articles retrieved from the total number of articles in the database.
- Recall or sensitivity is defined as the proportion of relevant articles retrieved from the total number of relevant articles in the database.

Dickersin et al (1995) discuss the factors which affect precision and recall, pointing out that the accuracy and completeness of the results depend largely on the quality of the search. Their test search found that sensitivity in MEDLINE, or recall of the number of relevant articles from a 'gold standard' total number of relevant articles, was 77%. Thus, even a trained searcher in MEDLINE did not retrieve everything that was available!

Stage 3 is particularly useful in three situations.

a. Too many references retrieved

Every searcher will have an opinion on what constitutes too many references. It can be defined only as being more references than a searcher wishes or feels it feasible to scan. The problem can occur if the search is too general. If you cannot define the subject more specifically, try the following options:

- Use the broad heading and do not explode it to exclude more specific aspects, e.g. benzodiazepines rather than all the individual drugs.
- Add a methodological term such as a review to find general articles that have looked at the literature.
- Restrict the search to articles published in the last few years.
- Limit the search to research articles that have abstracts, excluding editorials etc. Exclude words in the abstract, then any free textwords. If all else fails, concentrate on words in the title alone.

b. Too few references retrieved

In many cases a zero result means it is necessary to go back to the planning stage to think of alternative terms. Try the following options:

- Look at the full record of a relevant reference to see how it has been indexed. The abstract may also give other ideas for synonyms.
- Most systems nowadays will attempt to compensate for variations in British and American spelling but make sure that all possibilities have been covered.
- Broaden the subject to include more general terms as well as specific elements, e.g. benzodiazepines and all the individual drugs.

However, if a trawl of several databases and all possibilities of words does not yield much, it could be that little has been written.

c. Few of the references are relevant

- This might happen if textwords are truncated too early. 'Nurs$' will include 'nursing' as well as 'nurse', 'nurses' and 'nursed'.
- Some reversal of the subject may also occur. General practitioners AND asthma will bring up asthma treated by general practitioners but also could include asthma in general practitioners.
- Beware of acronyms and homonyms. BDA can stand for the British Dental Association or the British Diabetic Association. The word 'environment' might mean the green fields of nature or an office work space.

A note on time and cost

Despite the detail of these guidelines, planning and executing a search does not require hours of time. From start to finish the whole process might take between 15 and 30 minutes. As planning the strategy does not require access to a database, it does not have to be followed immediately by the search. However, the merit in seeing the whole process through at one sitting lies in the concentration of your thoughts. The earlier a strategy is planned in advance of the search, the more time will be required to refocus thoughts in implementing the search. The length of time involved depends on the complexity of the question, which database is being searched and the skills of the searcher. If the results are not satisfactory, it is worth spending 10 minutes reviewing the strategy.

The costs involved in searching are difficult to detail. Much of these will depend on the database being searched and the method of access. If you access MEDLINE through the BMA library, the cost should be the length of the telephone call. However, since MEDLINE is not a full-text database, further costs may be incurred in obtaining copies of the articles retrieved by the search. These costs vary enormously between libraries and can only be determined at the point of use. Searching databases over the Internet may also incur costs, but again this should be the cost of a telephone call — assuming that you are already paying a subscription to an Internet provider.

Conclusion

This chapter has focused on the process of conducting a literature search. It is a guide to the three stages of searching, and by following the steps through planning the strategy, implementing the search and evaluating the results you are equipped to try searching the literature for yourself. These stages do not guarantee 100% success. Although the method is logical to a certain extent, progressing from the initial idea through to execution of a planned strategy, literature searching can be as much of an art as it is a science. From a personal point of view, the best searches are conducted with a mixture of method and intuition. In fact it sometimes seems to be the case that the greater the degree of intuition used, the more satisfactory the search becomes. The last guideline to add is be prepared to regroup your thoughts and consider the possibility that perhaps there is no exact answer to your question in the current literature.

References

Dickersin K, Scherer R, Lefebvre C 1995 Identifying relevant studies for systematic reviews. In: Chalmers I, Altman D G (eds) Systematic reviews. British Medical Journal Publishing, London, pp 17–36

Kiley R 1996 Medical information on the Internet: a guide for health professionals. Churchill Livingstone, Edinburgh

Lee N, Millman A 1996 ABC of medical computing. British Medical Journal Publishing, London

Lefebvre C 1994 The Cochrane Collaboration: the role of the UK Cochrane Centre in identifying the evidence. Health Libraries Review 11:235–242

Lowe H J, Barnett G O 1994 Understanding and using the Medical Subject Headings (MeSH) vocabulary to perform literature searches. Journal of the American Medical Association 271:1103–1108

CHAPTER 3

What are parents' worries when their child has an acute illness?
An approach to evidence from qualitative research

Myfanwy Morgan and Leone Ridsdale

The clinical problem

On Saturday evening one of us (LR) was doing the evening base surgery for the GP cooperative. Patients brought their medical emergencies to the base surgery; bedbound patients and those with no car were visited by a second doctor in a car. As the practice had a new trainee (Dr J), he came too and we discussed the patients' problems.

The first patient was a 1-year-old boy brought in by both his parents who seemed very concerned. They said that their baby had run a high temperature for the past 24 hours, and that he seemed to be 'burning up'. LR asked if this was their first child and they confirmed that he was.

The second patient was a boy of 4 years who came with his mother. She had found a rash whilst bathing him, and was worried that it might be meningitis.

Three-quarters of the patients seen in the base surgery were children with acute infections. The trainee remarked that the Saturday evening surgery was very similar to his usual morning surgeries in terms of the minor problems seen. LR suggested that he look at the literature on parents' concerns about acute illness in their children. Dr J found a paper by Kai (1996a), published in the *British Medical Journal* with the title, 'What worries parents when their preschool children are acutely ill, and why: a qualitative study'. This paper (see pp 44–51) appeared to address his question directly. However, Dr J knew little about qualitative research. Moreover, he had occasionally heard qualitative research being dismissed for being 'anecdotal' and/or 'unscientific', because it does not adopt the same procedures of sampling or measurement as experimental or other 'quantitative' research. For example, qualitative studies usually involve relatively small numbers of subjects, and data comprise verbatim interview material or descriptions of observations rather than more familiar numerical data. Such studies are therefore occasionally viewed by clinical researchers as merely an assembly of anecdotes and personal impressions, which are not reproducible or generalizable. However, Dr J had seen the purposes and methods of qualitative research discussed in the medical literature. This included a series of seven articles in the *British Medical Journal* (reprinted as a BMJ book by Mays & Pope (eds) 1996), and papers published in *Family Practice* (Britten et al 1995; Hamberg et al 1994; Malterud 1993) and *Quality in Health Care* (Fitzpatrick & Boulton 1994). He was interested to learn more about qualitative methods and their application in Kai's study. Dr J decided to discuss this with a social scientist (MM) at his local medical school. The first question they considered was why a qualitative design was selected for this research.

Rationale for a qualitative study

The choice of research methods depends on the research question one wants to address, as the methods provide access to different types of knowledge (Pill 1995). Quantitative and qualitative methods thus contribute in different ways to the practice of evidence-based medicine and the process of patient care (Greenhalgh 1996; Murphy & Mattson 1992).

Quantitative survey-based studies are concerned with establishing statistical associations between variables. This design is therefore appropriate if, for example, one wishes to test whether use of general practitioner services when a child is acutely ill is related to the mother's own psychological health (Leach et al, 1993), or to examine the influence of various patient and practice characteristics on the use of general practitioners' out-of-hours care (Majeed et al, 1995). Qualitative methods are generally more appropriate if the primary aim, as in the present study, is to *understand* the beliefs and meanings that guide people's behaviours, or to investigate complex social processes. They are also particularly suitable for identifying the important issues and dimensions in relation to a relatively unexplored topic, as in the case of parents' worries about an acutely ill child. This is because rather than specifying relevant variables and dimensions in advance, a qualitative approach acknowledges that parents' own meanings may differ in important ways from the assumptions of doctors or

Table 3.1 Criteria for assessing qualitative research evidence

1. Is a qualitative approach appropriate for the questions being asked?
2. Is there a clear and well-justified account of the sampling strategy and is it appropriate?
3. Does it appear that the methods of data collection were sensitive to the research question and that possible sources of bias have been considered?
4. Is the research process clearly described, with all relevant information about the setting and subjects supplied?
5. Were the data analysed in a systematic way, with an emphasis on conceptual development?
6. Are the data presented in a systematic way which demonstrates the relationship between the evidence and the conclusions drawn?
7. Was there an attempt to test the validity of the findings?
8. Do the findings seem credible and generalizable?

researchers, and thus seeks to elicit respondents' own accounts in relatively open interviews.

The appraisal of a qualitative study is based on the general principles of good research practice and requires that the processes of data collection, data analysis and interpretation are systematic and rigorous, and are clearly described (see Table 3.1). Moreover, the aim of qualitative studies is to produce a plausible and coherent explanation of the phenomena under scrutiny which is 'generalizable' or transferable to other similar contexts. The main difference between qualitative and other types of research is in the methods adopted in relation to different aspects of the research process. Dr J therefore examined how the various stages of the research had been conducted and whether these conformed with good practice.

How were the data collected?

Two methods of data collection were employed: one-to-one interviews with parents and focus group discussions. Personal interviews are the most common method of data collection in qualitative research. However, they differ from interviews in quantitative research in being less structured and more flexible. Rather than consisting of a series of structured questions with predefined multiple choice answers, respondents in qualitative research studies are encouraged to describe and discuss their beliefs and behaviours in their own words. This is because a fundamental requirement of this research approach is that the participants' own perspective of the phenomenon of interest should unfold. The interviewers' questions are therefore adapted to follow the flow of the interview, and responses are gently probed and clarified as required so that views are fully described and the meanings and context are clear. Thus Kai describes how the interviews explored broad areas identified in a pilot study, but also concentrated on encouraging parents to discuss freely what was important to them when coping with ill young children and how and why they thought as they did. He described this approach as 'semi-structured', in contrast to an 'unstructured' or 'in-depth' interview. The latter terms refer to interviews in which the respondent is encouraged to talk as fully and freely as possible about one or two topics of interest, and is less directed by the interviewer (Britten 1996). However, the distinction between different types of interview is not clear-cut because interviews in qualitative research always involve a flexible agenda and take the form of a guided conversation in contrast to the more formal structured interview of quantitative research. The term 'in-depth' is therefore frequently applied as a general term to interviews in qualitative research.

Focus group interviews were used to complement the personal interviews. This refers to holding group discussions on a topic or series of issues which are conducted by a trained facilitator (Barbour 1995; Kitzinger 1996). Focus groups were originally used in communication studies to explore the effects of films and television programmes and have formed an important tool in marketing research. They are now increasingly employed in the health field to develop health promotion materials, to identify public priorities and concerns in relation to health services, and to explore the attitudes and needs of both patients and staff. The conduct of focus groups differs in the extent to which the researcher guides discussion and aims to cover a list of questions, or takes a more open respondent-led approach, as appears to have occurred in the present study. However, the general rationale for a focus group is that people are encouraged to talk to one another, ask questions, exchange anecdotes and comment on each other's experiences and points of view. These group processes can have the advantage of helping people to explore and clarify their views in ways that are less easily accessible in a one-to-one interview. They also allow participants to discuss issues of importance to them in their own vocabulary, to generate their own questions and pursue their own priorities. They are therefore useful in examining not only what people think, but also how they think and why they think as they do. In addition, the process of group discussion and interaction may serve to highlight (sub)cultural values or group norms that are often not tapped through personal interviews. As Kitzinger (1996) says, 'Focus groups reach the parts that other methods cannot reach.' However, although the dynamics of such groups can make positive contributions, their negative aspects are that the articulation of group norms may silence individual voices of dissent. In addition, the presence of other participants compromises the confidentiality of the research session and may inhibit some disclosures. The focus groups in the present study, however, are unlikely to have been constrained by such problems, as participants were all drawn from parents attending three parent and toddler groups, which meant that they had much in common and knew each other. The topic discussion was also personally non-threatening and one of which all mothers are likely to have had experience, thus encouraging full participation and interaction. In addition, this formed just one method of data collection and was complemented by personal interviews.

Who were the subjects and how were they selected?

An important consideration in guiding the design of the present study was Kai's decision to focus on parents (mainly mothers) with a young child (under 5 years old) living in a 'disadvantaged' area. This is because, as he notes in the introduction, children from disadvantaged backgrounds have the highest GP consultation rates and highest prevalence of morbidity. However, Dr J felt it would have been useful for this focus to have been apparent from the title.

Random sampling is sometimes employed to select subjects for qualitative research. However, in this study the procedure of 'purposeful' sampling was employed to select parents for interview, with the aim of ensuring that they included the variety of experiences and worries among such parents, and that the study group was therefore comprehensive and representative in these terms. Parents were therefore recruited from different community settings that were likely to include large numbers of relatively disadvantaged parents with a young child. These comprised a community centre, a hostel for single mothers, an inner city general practice, and three parent and toddler groups. Parents attending the community centre and parents living in the hostel were invited by the community worker to participate in the research. In addition a random group of 1 in 4 mothers registered with the general practice were sent a postal invitation.

Qualitative studies are generally based on fairly small numbers of subjects. This is because the aim is to undertake an in-depth investigation of people's beliefs and meanings and to achieve generalizable concepts, categories or explanations, rather than to establish the prevalence of particular variables. However, the precise numbers and methods of recruitment in qualitative research vary according to the specific aims of the research and broader aspects of the study design.

Kai did not set a predetermined number of interviews at the outset. Instead he continued interviewing until no new concepts were being generated, which suggested that the data set was comprehensive. The precise criteria he adopted for selecting parents for interview is, however, not entirely clear. He explains that, 'Initially, parents from each of the three settings (i.e. community centre, hostel and general practice) who might have had typical experiences (no specific characteristics) were interviewed. As the research progressed, I selected patients registered with the general practice who were thought to have particular experiences of caring for ill children and those who were thought to have atypical experiences after discussion with the practice.'

Altogether 28 mothers (4 with their male partners) were interviewed at home. Presentation of the key characteristics of the parents interviewed indicates that they comprised 4 single mothers of different ages in temporary hostel accommodation, 4 parents of children with chronic health problems (asthma, epilepsy), 3 parents of children with acute illness in the previous 12 months, 2 parents of children with special needs (Down's syndrome, tuberous sclerosis), 5 frequent users of general practitioner's out-of-hours service, 3 mothers with health professional backgrounds (2 nurses, 1 health service manager), and 7 others with preschool children. These characteristics thus suggest that the sample did encompass people with a range of experiences in terms of childhood health problems and were drawn from predominately disadvantaged backgrounds. The size of the interview group is fairly typical of qualitative research, which emphasizes the investigation of subjects' beliefs and worries in depth rather than quantification and statistical analysis. In addition, the personal interviews were complemented by 10 focus groups, with 5–8 mothers in each group.

Conducting the interviews

The interviews took between one and two hours. This relatively long length of interview is fairly typical of qualitative research, which requires issues to be examined in detail in an informal manner. Important influences on the data collected are how the subjects perceive the research, where it is conducted and their relationship with the researcher. Kai's paper does not make clear precisely what the parents were told about the research. However, we are informed that the one-to-one interviews were conducted in parents' homes and were thus on the respondents' own territory. This is important in encouraging a fuller discussion and greater disclosure of people's personally held beliefs than usually occurs when interviews are held on medical premises. However, Kai himself was the interviewer and, as he acknowledges, differences between himself (a male, middle-class health professional) and the respondents may have led them to exclude views that they believed might be considered unacceptable to a health professional. This potential source of bias was reduced by not including his own practice patients in the main sample, and because the topic under discussion was not of a particularly sensitive or threatening nature. In addition, a single interviewer/researcher both eliminates problems of possible interviewer variability and ensures the researcher is familiar with the context of the data, which aids interpretation. Different approaches thus each carry their potential advantages and limitations, while the methodological discussion in the paper shows the author was aware of and sensitive to these issues.

How were the data analysed?

Both the interviews and group discussions were audiotaped and transcribed in full. This allows the interviewer to listen attentively and respond without the interference of note-taking, and for a complete transcript of the interview to be available for analysis. Rather than involving statistical procedures to identify associations and relationships, data analysis in qualitative research is non-numeric and involves the analysis of text to derive concepts and explanations based on the respondents' own meanings. The present paper does not describe this process of analysis in detail but states that it was based on the procedures of 'grounded theory' (Strauss & Corbin 1990). This term is frequently employed to describe all qualitative analyses which follow the general procedures of conceptual development. This requires that preliminary concepts and categories are tested in relation to all cases, and as a result are modified or discarded until a stage is reached when the conceptual scheme fits the data. However, a specific feature of a grounded theory approach employed in this study was that data collection and analysis proceeded at the same time, with new data thus serving to test emerging concepts. The process of data collection therefore continued until no new ideas or categories were suggested by further data collection, rather than meeting a predetermined target.

The analysis of qualitative data is time-consuming and places considerable demands on the researcher. It requires a thorough familiarity with the data, as well as the systematic testing of concepts and relationships in a process of conceptual analysis (Fitzpatrick & Boulton 1994). Computer software programs are now frequently employed to assist with handling the large quantity of non-numeric data and allow textual analysis to be more systematic. For example, these programs enable researchers to organize and access their data by searching large amounts of text for specific terms, to define variables that can be used for selective retrieval and to examine links between different parts of the data (Fielding & Lee (eds) 1991). Kai provides little description of the actual process of analysis, but he appears to have relied on a traditional manual approach, which makes it difficult to examine all cases systematically in relation to emerging constructs. However, even when computer software is employed, its role is limited to facilitating access to the material. Interpretation and conceptual development necessarily rely on the researcher deriving meanings, and testing emerging explanations and categories in relation to the data.

What are the findings?

Fever, cough and the possibility of meningitis consistently emerged as parents' primary concerns when their children became acutely ill. These provoked particular anxiety because of fears that their child would die or be irreparably harmed. Each type of worry and the reasons for parents' particular responses to their child's illness are illustrated with verbatim quotations, although the relatively short length of a medical compared with a social science article limits the presentation of detailed case material. The data collected in interviews and focus groups leads Kai to develop an explanatory scheme of parents' management of ill children (see Fig. 1, p. 47). This depicts parents' anxieties about fever and cough as depending on two key factors. One of these was parents' perception of the risk or threat posed by the problem. This in turn was influenced by parents' perception of behavioural changes, such as their child not eating or sleeping, or not being herself or himself; their child being uncomfortable, such as hurting from coughing or flushing from fever; and if they thought their child was suffering, for example, from the physical effects of fever or from difficulty in breathing because of coughing. At this stage parents often worried that the problem might herald more severe illness or potential harm. In the case of fever this included worries about the development of meningitis or fits; permanent impairment of some kind, such as brain damage; or even death. A fever without other common signs of illness, and therefore an explanation (such as a cold), was described as being especially likely to cause concern and vigilance. In addition, for some parents a rising fever posed a more intangible, ill-defined threat. Coughs that were perceived as 'chesty' due to phlegm or that provoked vomiting or retching caused concern about infection 'on the chest'. Some feared development of a more chronic problem such as asthma or worried about the death of their child.

The second factor identified as shaping parents' responses was how they perceived their own ability to control symptoms and protect their child from potential harm. This involved attempting to reduce the fever and avoiding what they feared: their child's temperature rising out of control and increasing risks of harm. This may reflect professional advice about the need to cool children regularly, particularly in relation to febrile fits, although the main purpose of this advice is to keep the child comfortable rather than being preventive. Parents also tried to reduce the effects of cough, particularly at night when the child was seen as more vulnerable and difficult to monitor, and they felt especially powerless when they failed to keep a problem under control and the perceived threat increased (see Fig. 1, p. 47). In addition, they worried about failing to recognize a serious problem such as meningitis, or missing something.

Kai thus depicts parents as experiencing considerable worries and as continuously assessing and reassessing their child's symptoms. Worries about their child often led to the need to share responsibility with others within their lay network or to seek professional advice. Some parents felt guilty about bothering their doctor but thought they had little choice. This was especially the case if their child had a rash, as this frequently caused them to worry about meningitis. It appeared that for many parents any unexplained rash could herald immediate danger and the need to seek medical advice. As Kai notes, parents' anxieties about meningitis must be interpreted in the light of recent media coverage and campaigns about the illness, and are intensified by such messages as, 'knowing the symptoms of meningitis could mean the difference between life and death'. In a companion paper published in the same issue of the *British Medical Journal* (Kai 1996b), he draws on the same data set to consider the particular difficulties parents have in understanding the doctor's assessment or actions, and reconciling this with their own views and observations regarding their child's illness. This included what parents perceived as the dismissal of an illness as a 'virus' with little further information, what appeared to them to be unexplained variations in whether antibiotics were prescribed, and insufficient advice about the management of common symptoms. As a result, parents did not feel empowered in understanding and coping with their child's illness and continued to worry.

Assessing the evidence

Dr J was interested to learn of the specific requirements and process of qualitative research, including the demands in terms of data collection and analysis that are presented by what at first may seem a relatively small in-depth study. Examination of the methods employed by Kai indicates that these were generally clearly described and conformed with the requirements of qualitative research. The main area of uncertainty was whether his position as a male doctor may have influenced parents' responses. However, central to establishing the validity of qualitative research is determining whether the constructs and explanations derived from the data are valid, and thus accurately reflect the subjects' meanings and interpretations. This was examined directly through the procedure of 'respondent validation', which is a well-recognized method of assessing validity in qualitative research. This was undertaken by holding three further focus groups to feed back and review the 'findings', in terms of the constructs and explanations developed by the researcher. Kai reports that these seemed to be true to the respondents' experiences, with the focus group discussions confirming rather than modifying the analysis.

A key question is, how common are the particular concerns identified by Kai? Qualitative studies based on random samples are able to provide an indication of the frequency with which particular beliefs, experiences or views occurred among their study group (Silverman 1987), although precise quantification requires larger representative samples. However, as the present study was based on a purposive rather than a representative random sample, it is not possible to assess the frequency with which views were held. Instead, the main contribution of the research is to provide an understanding of why parents consult when their child is acutely ill in situations where doctors do not regard this as necessary, and to provide a clear understanding of the particular worries and anxieties that result in such consultations and thus of the demands placed on medical professionals' time.

Returning to the problem

Having found a paper on parents' concerns and appraised the evidence, LR and Dr J reflected on their experience of working in the base surgery. The concerns that we observed among parents were similar to those identified by Kai in a disadvantaged area. Knowing that these fears are so common, Dr J decided that in future he would enquire systematically about them when parents presented a child with an acute infection. The information he provided could then be targeted towards the parents' specific fears. For example, if they were frightened that their child seemed to be burning up, they could be reassured that the fever itself would be unlikely to harm the child. If parents were worried about losing control, the doctor might enquire about how they were managing and what they had already done. If it was possible, the doctor could then reassure them that they were doing the appropriate things to take care of their child and make him or her comfortable.

> **Returning to the problem** *(cont'd)*
>
> The findings in the paper are consistent with the experience of LR as a GP. When doctors learn about the fears of their patients, sometimes that a childhood illness like cough could lead to sudden death, they understand that what may seem a trivial complaint from a medical perspective was, from the point of view of a worried parent, vitally important (Cornford et al, 1993). Patients, or parents, often need specific reassurance from someone, who may be a grandmother, a friend, or for those without a supportive network, a doctor or nurse. In addition, there is often a need for health education to give parents more detailed information and for doctors to explain more fully. This should enable parents to feel more confident and, for example, help them to decide whether a rash may be meningitis, or know why they may be advised to cool a child with fever. More generally, Dr J felt that having a better understanding of parents' concerns would help him communicate more effectively when they consulted with an acutely ill child.

References

Barbour R S 1995 Using focus groups in general practice research. Family Practice 12: 328–334

Britten N 1996 Qualitative interviews in medical research 4. In: Mays N, Pope C (eds) Qualitative research in health care. British Medical Journal Publishing, London

Britten N, Jones R, Murphy E, Stacy R 1995 Qualitative research methods in general practice and primary care. Family Practice 12: 104–114

Cornford C, Morgan M, Ridsdale L 1993 Why do mothers consult when their children cough? Family Practice 10: 193–196

Fielding N, Lee R (eds) 1991 Using computers in qualitative research. Sage, London

Fitzpatrick R, Boulton M 1994 Qualitative methods for assessing health care. Quality in Health Care 3: 107–113

Greenhalgh T 1996 Is my practice evidence-based? British Medical Journal 313: 957–958

Hamberg K, Johansson E, Lingren G, Westman G 1994 Scientific rigour in qualitative research — examples from a study of women's health in family practice. Family Practice 11: 176–181

Kai J 1996a What worries parents when their preschool children are acutely ill, and why: a qualitative study. British Medical Journal 313: 983–986

Kai J 1996b Parents' difficulties and information needs in coping with acute illness in preschool children: a qualitative study. British Medical Journal 313: 987–990

Kitzinger J 1996 Introducing focus groups. In: Mays N, Pope C (eds) Qualitative research in health care. British Medical Journal Publishing, London, ch 5

Leach J, Ridsdale L, Smeeton N 1993 Is there a relationship between a mother's mental state and consulting the doctor by the family? Family Practice 10: 305–311

Majeed F A, Cook D G, Hilton S, Poloniecki J, Hagen A 1995 Annual night visiting rates in 129 general practices in one family health services authority: association with patient and general practice characteristics. British Journal of General Practice 45: 531–535

Malterud K 1993 Shared understanding of the qualitative research process: guidelines for the medical researcher. Family Practice 10: 201–206

Mays N, Pope C (eds) 1996 Qualitative research in health care. British Medical Journal Publishing, London

Murphy E, Mattson B 1992 Qualitative research and family practice: a marriage made in heaven? Family Practice 9(1): 85–91

Pill R 1995 Fitting the method to the question: the quantitative or qualitative approach? In: Jones R, Kinmouth A L (eds) Critical reading for primary care. Oxford University Press, Oxford

Silverman D 1987 Communication and medical practice. Sage, London

Strauss A, Corbin J 1990 Basics of qualitative research: grounded theory procedures and techniques. Sage, London

© British Medical Journal 1996; **313**: 983–6

What worries parents when their preschool children are acutely ill, and why: a qualitative study

Joe Kai

Abstract

Objective — To identify and explore parents' concerns when young children become acutely ill.
Design — Qualitative study making use of semistructured one to one and group interviews with parents of preschool children.
Setting — Disadvantaged inner city community.
Subjects — 95 parents of preschool children.
Results — Fever, cough, and the possibility of meningitis were parents' primary concerns when their children became acutely ill. Parents' concerns reflected lay beliefs, their interpretation of medical knowledge, and their fears that their child might die or be permanently harmed. Parents worried about failing to recognise a serious problem. Concerns were expressed within the context of keenly felt pressure, emphasising parents' responsibility to protect their child from harm. They were grounded in two linked factors: parents' sense of personal control when faced with illness in their child and the perceived threat posed by an illness.
Conclusions — Better understanding of parents' concerns may promote effective communication between health professionals and parents. Modification of parents' personal control and perceived threat using appropriate information and education that acknowledge and address their concerns may be a means of empowering parents.

Introduction

Children under 5 years old form the largest proportion of reactive workload in primary care, with those from disadvantaged backgrounds having the highest contact rates and morbidity.[4] Parents inevitably worry about their children when they are ill. Gaining an understanding of what parents worry about is important if parents' anxieties are to be addressed effectively and if relevant information and education is to be offered. Previous work has described the beliefs and behaviours of mothers with young children but has paid less attention to what provokes concern for parents when their children are acutely ill. In this study and the accompanying paper[9] I sought to identify what worries parents when their children become acutely ill and to understand what motivates their concerns.

Subjects and methods

I conducted pilot interviews initially with parents who were patients registered on the shared list of my general practice. I then recruited parents who were not my patients and had at least one child under 5 years old from a range of community settings in a disadvantaged area: a community centre, a hostel for single mothers, another inner city general practice, and three parent and toddler groups.

One to one interviews   Parents attending the community centre and parents living in the hostel were invited to participate in the

Department of Primary Health Care, Medical School, University of Newcastle upon Tyne, Newcastle upon Tyne NE2 4HH Joe Kai, *lecturer in primary health care*

Continued →

research by a community worker. A random one in four sample of mothers registered with the general practice was sent a postal invitation. Purposeful sampling[10,11] was then used to select willing parents for interview. Initially, parents from each of the three settings who might have had typical experiences (no specific characteristics) were interviewed. As the research progressed, I selected parents registered with the general practice who were thought to have particular experiences of caring for ill children and those who were thought to have atypical experiences after discussion with the practice. Such parents were actively sought to ensure that data and its interpretation were not distorted to one perspective and that all cases could be accommodated within the developing analysis. Sampling was intended to provide a range of experiences and perceptions so that the breadth of findings and concepts emerging might be understood. Table 1 describes those features of the resulting sample. The interviews were open ended, semi-structured, and conducted in parents' homes.

Focus group interviews All parents attending three parent and toddler groups were invited by their group organisers to form a volunteer sample to participate in focus group interviews.[12] These were held where they usually met with the help of creche facilities. Both one to one and group interviews were used to enhance the sufficiency and quality of data and facilitate comparison and confirmation of emerging concepts across different settings.

Data analysis The interviews explored broad areas identified in the pilot but concentrated on encouraging parents to discuss freely what was important to them when coping with ill young children and how and why they thought as they did. All interviews were audiotaped and transcribed

verbatim. Data collection and analysis were guided by grounded theory methodology. Transcriptions were analysed to identify concepts and categories embedded within them. Concepts and their relations were confirmed, modified, or discarded from ongoing analysis by re-examination of earlier data and during subsequent data collection and analysis. Interviewing continued until no new concepts were being generated. This suggested that the findings and conceptual scheme developed were a valid picture of parents' concerns and perceptions.

Study sample Ninety five parents were interviewed in total. Of parents invited to participate in the one to one interviews, 16 of the 22 mothers at the community centre, all four parents at the hostel, and 29 of the 47 mothers registered with the general practice

Table 1 Purposeful sample of parents in one to one interviews

Key characteristics of family interviewed	No of mothers (n=28)
Single mother in temporary hostel accommodation	4*
Child with chronic problems (asthma, epilepsy)	4
Child admitted with acute illness in previous 12 months	3
Child with special needs (Down's syndrome, tuberous sclerosis)	2
Frequent user of general practitioner's out of hours service	5†
Mother with health professional background	3‡
Others with preschool child or children	7

*Two aged 16, one aged 18, one aged 25
†Two or more out of hours visits by general practitioner to all children under 5 years old in past 12 months
‡One auxiliary nurse, one registered general nurse, one health service manager (sample included four fathers)

Continued →

Table 2 Characteristics of participants

	No of households (n=91)
Unemployed household*	34
Living in rented housing	58
Mother left full time education at 16 or under	64
Mother without formal qualifications since leaving school†	54
Single parent household	29
Household with one child	31

*No parent in employment.
†Educational or vocational.

agreed. Ultimately, 32 parents were selected and interviewed at home (24 mothers alone and four mothers with their male partners). A further 63 mothers (of 82 attending the parent and toddler groups) participated in 10 focus groups (range 5–8 mothers). All the interviews lasted between one and two hours and were conducted over a period of 14 months. Most parents were from socioeconomically disadvantaged backgrounds. All were white and English speaking. The mean age of mothers was 26 years (range 16–41 years). The characteristics of participants are summarised in tables 1 and 2.

Respondent validation   To establish that the dataset was complete and parents' experiences were fully described, three further focus groups were held to feed back and review findings.[14] Nineteen parents, six who had been interviewed individually and 13 who had been part of a focus group, took part. The description and interpretation of the data seemed to be true to their experiences, the additional information from these discussions confirming rather than modifying the analysis.

Results

Fever, cough, and the possibility of

meningitis consistently emerged as parents' primary concerns when their children became acutely ill. These provoked particular anxiety because of fears that their child would die or be irreparably harmed. These concerns are discussed below to illustrate an explanatory scheme of parents' management of ill children developed through the analysis. Two key linked factors were involved: perceived threat and personal control. Other concerns and difficulties parents described are discussed in the accompanying paper.'

Perceived threat

Parents' anxieties about fever and cough, and the importance that they attached to them during an episode of illness, related to how parents interpreted their apparent effects on their child. This shaped their assessment of risk or the perceived threat posed by an illness. Of initial concern were changes in behaviour that parents associated with their child becoming unwell, such as not eating or sleeping or not being herself or himself. Parents became more concerned if their child was uncomfortable – for example, hurting from coughing or flushing from fever. They became more anxious if they thought their child was suffering – for example, from the physical effect of a fever or from difficulty in breathing because of coughing (box 1). At this stage parents often worried that the problem might herald more severe illness or potential harm. In the case of fever this included the development of meningitis or fits; permanent impairment of some kind, such as brain damage; or even death. A fever without other common signs of illness, and therefore an explanation (such as a cold), was especially likely to cause concern and vigilance. For some parents a rising fever posed a more intangible, ill defined threat (box 1).

Continued →

Box 1 Suffering and potential harm

Suffering
'I hate it when you see them like that, they're just burning up, lying there crying and not eating' (Parent 11)

'I worry about him getting chesty … he really can hardly breathe sometimes he's coughing that much' (Parent 5)

Potential harm
'When their temperature goes too high it's worrying, you worry about brain damage and things, and they could die, or there might be something more deeply worrying than I could imagine' (Parent 20)

Box 2 Managing the problem

'I always keep an eye on the temperature, I like to get their temperature down … that's the frightening stage when it keeps rising and rising' (Parent 23)

'He sounded like he was choking, I kept making sure he was okay during the night' (Parent 6)

'I panicked and called the doctor … she was choking and it was a horrible barking cough and she brought loads of phlegm up making her sick … there was nothing I could do … I thought she was going to die' (Parent 3, group 5)

Coughs that were perceived as 'chesty' due to phlegm or that provoked vomiting or retching caused concern about infection 'on the chest.' Some feared development of a more chronic problem such as asthma or worried about death of their child from the sudden infant death syndrome, from inhaling vomit, or, more usually, from choking. Perceived

threat, then, comprised categories reflecting the observed effects of a problem and beliefs about the potential harm that might result (Fig. 1).

Personal control

Monitoring and maintaining control of symptoms was seen as paramount to

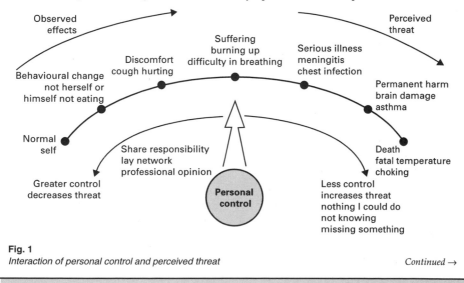

Fig. 1
Interaction of personal control and perceived threat

Continued →

minimise discomfort and reduce the threat of harm. Parents continuously assessed their child's temperature (most often by touch) and diligently performed cooling procedures. They were preoccupied with the fever becoming too high: their common fear was of a temperature rising inexorably, eventually spiralling out of their control and bringing the threat of harm nearer. Management of cough entailed a similar process of checking and trying to reduce the effects of the cough, particularly at night when the child was seen as more vulnerable and difficult to monitor. Parents felt increasingly powerless when their efforts were failing to keep a problem under control and the perceived threat increased (box 2).

Analysis of parents' strategies showed that they watched, checked, and tried to make sense of their child's illness. At the heart of this lay an imperative responsibility to ensure the safety of their child. Parents expressed frustration at feeling ignorant, and they worried about failing to recognise a serious problem, about missing something (box 3). A parent's personal control encompassed her sense of being able to control the observed effects of an illness and to protect her child from potential harm. This was conditioned by her knowledge, beliefs, and experiences and informed her evaluation and management of a problem. Figure 1 depicts a model of the interaction of personal control regulating perceived threat.

> **Box 3** Lack of control
>
> 'If I knew what the problem was I don't think I'd be as worried, it's not knowing that gets to me' (Parent 16)
>
> 'When she's got a bug … I'm worried that it's something else, and I'm missing something … it could be something nasty … I don't know' (Parent 4)

The need to share responsibility with others within their lay network or by seeking professional advice could be irresistible when parents were concerned about their child. Some parents felt guilty about bothering their doctor in these circumstances but thought that they had little choice (box 4). These issues were foremost when parents talked about meningitis. Discussion about meningitis was often emotive. Parents' deepest fears of death or handicap befalling their child crystallised in the form of meningitis. There was a common understanding that symptoms could be non-specific and the illness rapidly overwhelming, heightening anxiety about not detecting the disease. For some parents the spectre of meningitis haunted them whenever their child showed signs of being more than slightly unwell (box 4). The specific feature of meningitis most often identified was appearance of a rash. Parents were ever vigilant for this sign of meningococcal illness, but few parents had accurate knowledge of the rash. For many parents any unexplained rash could herald immediate danger and the need to seek medical advice.

Discussion

Methodological considerations

This study has highlighted the primary concerns of parents when young children become acutely ill and has explored why they worry about them. A qualitative approach was used to provide insights into parents' concerns and thinking rather than produce statistically representative results. Most parents were willing to participate. I did not gather comprehensive information about non-respondents, however, as I did not want parents to feel uncomfortable or under pressure to participate when many had hectic schedules, particularly in the community

Continued →

Box 4 Sharing responsibility and meningitis fear

Sharing responsibility
Father: 'Once the doctor's been out and had a look you feel a lot easier in yourself'

Mother: 'You think, 'Am I phoning him up for nothing? ... but at the end of the day if you didn't and something happened to your baby you would never forgive yourself' (Parents 15A and B)

Spectre of meningitis
Parent 5: You don't really know what you're looking for do you?

Parent 6: No. I mean you hear about it on the telly and it starts from flu symptoms, things like that, and you think straight away they're not getting better, that's it, it must be meningitis

Parent 4: You always worry about meningitis ... in case you don't catch it quick enough

Parent 5: Well you get no symptoms at the beginning ... meningitis does not give any warning (Group 3)

centre and toddler groups. Moreover, I wanted a sample of parents who were willing to articulate their experiences.

The systematic methods described were used to increase the reliability and validity of the study: selecting a broad range of parents with different experiences; obtaining data in both one to one and group settings; and reviewing and confirming the findings with participants themselves. In the focus groups parents were already familiar with each other. This may have reduced the artificiality of the discussions. These groups explored one of the social contexts in which ideas might be formed and decisions made about young children's illness. Conversely, respondent validation used discussions between previously interviewed participants who were not known to each other and allowed comparison of parents' experiences in another context.

Differences between the researcher and respondents may have influenced parents' responses and their interpretation: I am a male middle class health professional and the respondents were largely women from disadvantaged backgrounds. Parents' public accounts may have been selective and excluded that which might be considered unacceptable to a health professional. Participants were aware that I was a doctor and discussion may have been biased towards medical rather than lay concepts. However, the study has attempted to place emphasis on the perceptions of the parents interviewed. I was also able to identify with some of the respondents' experiences as I have worked as a general practitioner in their community for the past five years. Few fathers were interviewed – the study reflects the contemporary reality of childcare, which remains largely the responsibility of mothers.

Understanding parents' concerns

When parents' concerns were explored, two factors emerged that appeared fundamental in shaping their responses: parents' sense of personal control when faced with illness in their child and the perceived threat posed by an illness. Germane to personal control was parents' experience of comparative ignorance and difficulty in establishing the severity of illness, which is discussed further in the accompanying paper. Parents' concerns were expressed within the context of keenly felt

Continued →

pressure to protect their child from harm. The perceived threat could be seen as a continuous process corresponding to the effects a problem was believed or observed to cause and regulated by a parent's personal control (Fig 1). This scheme has resonance with the folk model of illness beliefs proposed by Helman. For example, fever was perceived as serious and its development outside personal control (thus requiring professional advice) in contrast to a common cold, in which the elements of personal responsibility and control are strong, its development being influenced by things such as not wrapping up well.

Parents' concerns about fever and cough reflected erroneous beliefs and use of biomedical concepts, albeit in a rational framework. Beliefs about fever rising relentlessly and the need to control temperature may be viewed as logical and congruent with fairly common knowledge of febrile convulsions and delirium in young children. In addition, advice from professionals commonly reinforces cooling children regularly, particularly in relation to febrile fits. However, controlling temperature is not necessarily preventive – the main purpose is to keep the child comfortable. Quantitative research from North America has pointed to similar beliefs. Parents may benefit from education about the probable positive effects of fever and the body's central regulatory thermostat.

The depth and nature of parents' concerns about cough accord with the high proportion of consultations for children in general practice that are for respiratory illness. Similar beliefs have been described among mothers who recently consulted a general practitioner about their child's cough.[20] The qualitative construction of perceived threat in the current study is also consistent with the characteristics of a child's cough which have been found to predict likelihood of consulting a general practitioner.[21] Increasing parents' knowledge of the nature of upper and lower respiratory tract infections and the physiological function of cough in response to infection may be helpful.

Parents' anxieties about meningitis must be interpreted in the light of recent media coverage and campaigns about the illness. The pressure parents experienced may have been intensified by messages such as 'knowing the symptoms of meningitis could mean the difference between life and death.'[22] Parents readily identified the need to be vigilant for a rash, yet self limiting rashes are common in young children. This may be creating unnecessary anxiety and increased contacts with health services. It underlines the need for information to include good photographs to show how to distinguish the rash of meningococcal illness, such as those in the material produced by Meningitis Research.[23]

Parents' anxieties about failing to recognise a serious illness serve as a reminder that what constitutes common knowledge for doctors may not be readily accessible to parents.

Key messages

- When faced with acute illness in their children, parents' concerns were shaped by their sense of personal control and the perceived threat posed by an illness
- Parents worried about fever, cough, the possibility of meningitis, and failing to recognise a serious problem
- Better understanding of parents' concerns and what causes them may promote more effective communication between health professionals and parents

Continued →

What are parents' worries when their child has an acute illness?

Information and education that address parents' concerns may empower parents by influencing perceptions of threat posed by an illness and enhancing personal control. This forms the basis of a hypothesis for further exploration. The findings emphasise the importance of acknowledging and addressing parents' fears and beliefs if a consultation is to help the parent and not be regarded as inappropriate by the health professional. With much current activity in general practice focused on managing the rising demand for out of hours care,[24,25] this research highlights a source of mutual dissatisfaction between the parents of ill young children, who generate much of this workload, and their general practitioners. Better understanding of parents' concerns and what motivates them may promote more effective communication between health professionals and parents.

I thank the parents who took part; Sharon Denley, project secretary: the primary care team of Adelaide Medical Centre for support and encouragement; Ethel Street Surgery, Gladys MacFarlane, Marge Craig, and Karen Gelder for help in recruiting participants; and Pauline Pearson, Ann Crosland, Kevin Jones, Rosie Stacy, John Howie, and an anonymous referee for helpful comments.

Funding: Northern and Yorkshire Regional Health Authority.

Conflict of interest: None.

1. McCormick A, Fleming D, Charlton J 1995 Morbidity statistics from general practice: fourth national study, 1991–92, London: HMSO
2. Wilkin D, Hallam L, Leavey R, Metcalfe D 1987 Anatomy of urban general practice. London: Tavistock
3. Campion PD, Gabriel J 1984 Child consultation patterns in general practice; comparing 'high' and 'low' consulting families. BMJ 288: 1426–8
4. Spencer N, Logan S, Scholey S, Gentle S 1996 Deprivation and bronchiolitis. Arch Dis Child 74: 50–2
5. Blaxter M, Patterson E 1982 Mothers and daughters: a three generational study of health attitudes and behaviour. London: Heinemann
6. Spencer NJ 1984 Parents' recognition of the ill child. In: MacFarlane JA, ed. Progress in child health. Edinburgh: Churchill Livingstone, 100–11
7. Mayall B 1986 Keeping children healthy. London: Allen and Unwin
8. Cunningham-Burley S 1990 Mothers' beliefs about and perceptions of their children's illness. In: Cunningham-Burley S, McKegancy N, eds. Readings in medical sociology. London: Routledge, 85–109
9. Kaj J 1996 Parents' difficulties and information needs in coping with acute illness in preschool children: a qualitative study. BMJ 313: 987–90
10. Glaser BG, Strauss AI 1967 The discovery of grounded theory. New York: Aldine
11. Bogdan R C, Biklen SR 1982 Qualitative research for education; an introduction to theory and methods. Boston: Allyn and Bacon
12. Kreuger R 1988 Focus groups, a practical guide for applied research. London: Sage
13. Strauss A, Corbin J 1990 Basics of qualitative research. Grounded theory procedures and techniques. London: Sage
14. Mays N, Pope C 1995 Rigour and qualitative research. BMJ 311: 109–12
15. Helman C 1980 Feed a cold, starve a fever. In: Currer C, Stacey M, eds. Concepts of health, illness and disease: a comparative perspective. Leamington Spa: Berg
16. Stephenson T, Dunn K 1994 The febrile child. Maternal and Child Health 19: 128–32
17. Schmirr B D 1980 Fever phobia. Am J Dis Child 134: 176–81
18. Kramer M S, Naimark L, Leduc D G 1985 Parental fever phobia and its correlates. Paediatrics 75: 1110–3
19. Kluger N J 1991 The adaptive value of fever. In: Mackowiak P A, ed. Fever: basic mechanisms and management. New York: Raven Press
20. Cornford C S, Morgan M, Ridsdale L 1993 Why do mothers consult when their children cough? Fam Pract 10: 193–6
21. Wyke S, Hewison J, Russell I 1990 Respiratory illness in children: what makes parents decide to consult? J R Coll Gen Pract 40: 226–9
22. Department of Health 1994 Knowing about meningitis and septicaemia. London: DoH (Leaflet)
23. Meningitis Research 1994 What to do if you suspect meningitis. Bristol: Meningitis Research
24. Hallam L 1994 Primary medical care outside normal working hours: review of published work. BMJ 308: 249–53
25. Hurwitz B 1995 The new out of hours agreement for general practitioners. BMJ 311: 824–5
(Accepted 7 August 1996)

CHAPTER 4

How can we improve our diagnosis of back pain?
An approach to managing diagnostic uncertainty

Tim Lancaster and Anthony Harnden

The clinical problem

A 62-year-old man consulted, complaining of pain in the right upper quadrant of the abdomen, and some shortness of breath. He had a history of asthma and was an ex-smoker. An ultrasound of the right upper quadrant of the abdomen was normal, and review of his records showed a normal chest X-ray taken 12 months previously. His breathing improved with an increase in dose of his inhaled steroids. Over the next 3 weeks, he continued to complain of pain, and this became localized to his back. His weight remained stable. Full blood count and routine biochemistry were normal, and an erythrocyte sedimentation rate (ESR) was reported at 22 mm/hour. An X-ray of the lumbar and thoracic spine was reported as showing degenerative changes only.

He was treated with non-steroidal anti-inflammatory agents and codeine, and had reasonable pain control for several months. He then developed acute abdominal and back pain and was referred to casualty for a surgical opinion. The referral diagnosis was a possible dissecting abdominal aortic aneurysm (not excluded by the previous ultrasound). Surgical opinion was that the back was the source of pain and referral for an orthopaedic opinion was suggested. The patient was sent home, and an appointment arranged. He continued to have a great deal of pain and before the appointment could take place, the pain became so severe that he was admitted as an emergency to an orthopaedic bed. He died shortly after admission, and autopsy showed that he died of pulmonary complications of bronchial carcinoma with lytic metastases in the thoracic and lumbar spine.

Introduction

Learning to tolerate and manage uncertainty is one of the goals of training for general practice. A great deal of this uncertainty is related to diagnosis, and in most cases it is easily tolerated because the consequences of getting it wrong are unimportant (for example, is this patient's sore throat due to a virus or a bacterium?). Uncertainty is much more stressful when misdiagnosis may have serious consequences, and most of us make strenuous efforts to reduce it when we feel the probability of serious illness is high. Nevertheless, we sometimes get it wrong, and such times, though painful, offer an opportunity to learn. In this chapter, we describe how we tried to learn from such an experience using an evidence-based approach. (Although an actual clinical experience prompted our search, we have used a fictional patient in this chapter to protect confidentiality.)

What do we need to know?

After discussing the problem, we felt that diagnosis had been delayed. Although various older and wiser colleagues pointed out to us that earlier diagnosis would not have changed the outcome in a patient with metastatic cancer, we felt that we might have been able to control symptoms and manage psychosocial aspects better if we had worked out what was going on sooner. We then asked ourselves why an earlier diagnosis had not been made. We were uncertain that we had placed correct weight on the clinical findings and the investigation findings, and wondered whether we should have pressed earlier for further investigation. Though we were both aware that plain X-rays of the spine are not 'very good' for detecting cancer, we realized we had no idea exactly what value they had. We considered the normal X-ray to be the main factor in falsely reassuring us about our patient's diagnosis. We therefore formulated the question, using the four-part strategy recommended by Richardson and colleagues (Richardson et al 1995). The aim of formalizing the question is that it makes it easier to search for information, particularly when using electronic databases. Most questions can be thought of as having at least three parts: a patient, an intervention or exposure, and an outcome. It may be helpful to include a fourth element to the question (a comparison), since most interventions are evaluated in comparison to doing something else.

In a middle-aged man with back pain (the patient), to what extent do plain X-rays (the intervention or manoeuvre) change the probability that cancer (the clinical outcome) is present, in comparison to clinical findings (the comparison manoeuvre)?

The search

Having formulated our question, we visited the library to look for further information. Using the Webspirs program to access the Silver Platter version of MEDLINE, we typed in 'back pain' and asked the program to look for this term in its index. The program offered various MeSH terms to do with back pain, including 'back-pain-diagnosis'. This seemed to fit the bill so we searched on this term and came up with 563 entries – too many to browse through comfortably. We then asked the program to search for 'sensitivity or specificity', and to combine this with the previous search. This has been suggested to be the best strategy for finding studies of diagnostic tests on MEDLINE (McKibbon & Walker-Dilks 1994). This yielded eight studies, of which the following looked the most promising: What can the history and physical examination tell us about low back pain? (Deyo et al 1992). This article was part of a series called 'The rational clinical examination' which we had previously found helpful, and was in a journal (*Journal of the American Medical Association – JAMA*) which we knew was readily available in our local library. Having spent less than 5 minutes on the computer, we tracked down the article. This article seemed to provide what we needed in a table which showed the sensitivity and specificity of various findings for cancer as a cause of back pain. However, because of the focus of this article, no data were given on the value of investigations such as X-rays and blood tests. The data were drawn from an original study looking at diagnostic strategies for patients with cancer and back pain (Deyo & Diehl 1988). This was published in a less readily available journal (see pp. 64–76), and we had to order it through the library, setting our search back by a week.

Interestingly, this study had not turned up in our original search, despite being concerned with diagnosis of back pain, and quoting sensitivity and specificity. When we examined its MEDLINE entry, the terms 'sensitivity' and 'specificity' did not appear in the abstract or the keywords, despite being central to the methods of the paper! This reiterates the point that indexing often limits the value of MEDLINE, and other strategies may be necessary before the best evidence turns up.

Evaluating the evidence

Article finally in hand, we set out to appraise it critically. To help us with this we turned to the articles on interpreting diagnostic test results by Jaeschke and colleagues (Jaeschke et al 1994a, 1994b), published as part of a *JAMA* series entitled 'Users' guides to the medical literature'. We followed the three steps they suggest. Firstly, we set out to determine whether the study was valid (can we trust the results?). We then determined what the results were (does the study contain the information we are after?), and finally tried to apply them to our particular clinical problems (are the results clinically useful?).

Is the study valid?

Jaeschke and colleagues suggest two criteria for determining whether a study of a diagnostic test is likely to be valid.

1. Was there an independent, blind comparison with a reference standard?

The accuracy of a diagnostic test is best determined by comparing it to the true diagnosis, rather than to another diagnostic test, which may itself be imperfect. Sometimes very good reference standards exist. For example, tissue samples can usually provide a definitive diagnosis of cancer. At other times, it may be more difficult to determine whether the condition is truly present or not. For Alzheimer's disease, for example, there is no immediate method of confirming the diagnosis, and thereby judging the accuracy of a diagnostic test. Such assessments may have to await long-term clinical follow-up, or even autopsy data.

2. Did the patient sample include an appropriate spectrum of patients to whom the diagnostic test will be applied in clinical practice?

It is important that a test be shown to discriminate between people who do and do not have the disease in a sample of patients that is representative of typical clinical practice. A test that distinguishes severely affected individuals from completely healthy ones is not of much clinical use if it is unable to separate out people who truly have the condition from those who have something similar but not as serious. For example, while virtually all patients with temporal arteritis will have an ESR higher than a healthy university student, the value of that ESR in distinguishing people with this condition from individuals with infections, arthritis and other conditions that could be confused with temporal arteritis is much lower.

Deyo and Diehl's study (1988) set out to collect data prospectively on a consecutive series of patients attending a walk-in primary care clinic in Seattle. A total of 1975 patients were studied with an age range of 15–86, and over half were seeking medical care for back pain for the first time. Most had low back pain. Although not precisely comparable to patients with back pain seen in British general practice, we felt that the study sample was broadly representative of a primary care population, and that the tests were being applied to a reasonable spectrum of patients, so the second criterion was met. The validity of the reference standard was more difficult to judge. The authors determined whether cancer was the cause of pain by follow-up through the regional cancer registry at least 6 months after the first visit. In itself, this seemed reasonable: it seemed unlikely that a cancer causing back pain would not be diagnosed within 6 months, and provided follow-up was good, we could have confidence about their diagnostic status. However, follow-up was a problem. Since the population was, by definition, transitory (using episodic care rather than follow-up with a regular doctor), it was possible that some might have left the region and developed cancer. Although the authors noted that 75% of a subset of these patients had described the clinic as their only source of medical care, they could offer no reassurance about the completeness of follow-up. This was a potential problem in interpreting the results, but we did not consider it a fatal flaw. If anything, the effect of this bias would probably be to weaken the link between positive test results and diagnosis. Since we were interested in a negative test result, the bias probably would not affect the message we drew from the paper. We therefore read on.

What were the results?

Having determined that the study is likely to yield valid information, the next step in critical appraisal is to determine what the results of the study are. For diagnostic tests, this will mean that there is information that allows us to judge the accuracy of the test, or series of tests, in question. In this chapter, we will focus on a particular method of assessing the accuracy of a test known as likelihood ratios.

Although we often use diagnostic tests when we suspect (or perhaps even know) they will not change our thinking (for reassurance, for example), diagnostic tests are most helpful when they lead to a clinically significant change in our estimate of the probability of disease. All tests may be falsely positive or falsely negative. One way of gauging the accuracy of a test (the extent to which these incorrect results occur) is to calculate sensitivity (the proportion of people with the disease in whom the test is positive) and specificity (the proportion of people without the disease in whom the test is negative).

Sensitivity and specificity are helpful when evaluating how well a test performs compared to other tests. They are less helpful concepts for clinicians wondering how a particular test result relates to an individual patient. An alternative method is to calculate likelihood ratios. The likelihood ratio of a test is the ratio of the sensitivity to 1-specificity. It typically yields a number greater than 1 if the test increases the probability of disease, and less than 1 if it decreases the probability of disease. A likelihood ratio of 1 leads to no change in the probability of disease. The great advantage of likelihood ratios is that they can be directly related to an individual to allow an adjustment of our estimate of the probability of disease before and after the test. Although this can be done mathematically, it is much simpler and quicker to use a nomogram devised by Fagan (Fagan 1975) (see Fig. 4.1).

Let's take a hypothetical patient who is judged, from clinical findings, to have a probability of disease of 50%. She then undergoes a test which is positive with a likelihood ratio of 10. If we anchor our pretest probability on the left-hand axis of the nomogram, and run a line from there through the likelihood ratio (LR) of 10 on the central axis, we can read off the post-test probability of disease on the right axis. This probability is over 90%. Depending on the diagnosis in question, we may be happy to accept this as the working diagnosis. For example, we might be happy to anticoagulate for a possible deep venous thrombosis at this level of certainty, but before administering chemotherapy for cancer we would want even higher diagnostic certainty (for example, histological evidence). If, on the other hand, we take a patient in whom we judge the pretest probability of disease to be much lower, say 10%, then a positive result on the same test with an LR of 10 will lead to a post-test probability of only about 55% — too uncertain to make a management decision in cases where the consequences of misdiagnosis may be serious.

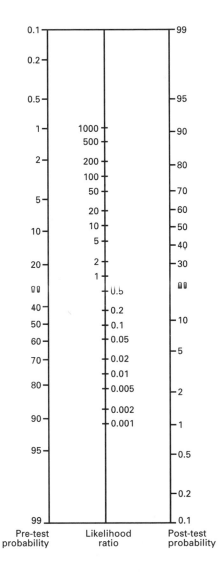

Fig. 4.1
Nomogram for interpreting diagnostic test results.
Adapted from Fagan T J 1975 Nomogram for Bayes's
therom. *New England Journal of Medicine* 293:257

In the paper by Deyo & Diehl (1988), not only was the
information necessary to calculate likelihood ratios given,
but the authors had also chosen this method to describe
their findings. The diagnostic value of clinical findings and
investigations are shown in Tables 2 and 3 of the paper on
pages 69 and 71.

Several clinical findings increased the likelihood of

cancer. The highest likelihood ratio (14.7) was associated with a previous history of cancer; the presence of this finding would therefore greatly increase the probability of cancer, raising a pretest probability of 50% to about 95%. Other findings which increased the likelihood of cancer to a smaller degree (LRs of 2–3) were unexplained weight loss, failure to improve after a previous visit in the past month, and age over 50. These findings would produce only modest shifts in probability. For example, they would change a pretest probability of 50% to a post-test probability of 60–70%.

Among test results, an ESR > 100 mmHg had a likelihood ratio of 55, while the presence of a lytic or blastic lesion on X-ray had a likelihood ratio of 120. Using the nomogram, we can show that the presence of either of these findings would greatly increase the probability that a serious cause for back pain was present whatever the pretest probability that cancer was present. In other words, a positive test would virtually rule in the diagnosis.

Will the results help me in caring for my patients?

Having found that the information we needed was available, we next set out to apply it to our patient. In order to use the results from the study, we first had to decide what the probability of cancer was in this patient before we tested. This, of course, is not a static estimate. Although we thought the probability of cancer was low, perhaps less than 5% at the first consultation, our estimate of this probability had risen as the patient made repeated visits to the surgery, and we thought that the probability of cancer was about 25%. Although we made this estimate 'intuitively', it is the shift in probability which would be predicted from Deyo's finding that failure to improve over time was associated with a likelihood ratio for cancer of 3.0. In other words, it is possible to quantify the clinical judgement of experienced doctors – an important point when we are trying to explain our judgements to students and others with less experience.

Having settled on this probability estimate from the clinical findings, we had to use the evidence to decide how a particular test result should change our estimate. We focused on the X-ray findings. As we have seen, the

presence of a lytic or blastic lesion is a powerful predictor of
the presence of cancer. In our case, however, the problem
was the reverse. We had a patient in whom our clinical
suspicion of serious disease was moderately large, but the
X-ray was 'negative'. The likelihood ratio of a normal X-ray
is calculated as (1-sensitivity/specificity), in this case
(0.4/0.995), giving a likelihood ratio of 0.4. Turning to the
nomogram, you can see how the meaning of this test result
varies depending on the pretest probability of disease. If our
clinical suspicion had been very low, say <5%, then a test
with a likelihood ratio of 0.4 would reduce the probability to
somewhere under 1%, which we might have been happy to
accept. In this case, however, our pretest probability that
there was a sinister cause for this man's back pain was about
25%. In this case, the 'normal' X-ray lowers the probability
of disease, but only to about 10% – not an acceptably low
figure to be confident that all was well. We therefore
concluded that our error in this case had been to attach too
much weight to the test result, and too little to our clinical
judgement. In the future, we have decided to bypass plain
X-rays altogether in this situation, and instead refer to a
specialist with a view to performing more sensitive
investigations.

When we have discussed this problem with students
and other colleagues, they sometimes object to placing a
number on the estimate for the pretest probability, arguing
that this confers an exactitude to what is quite a wide
range of uncertainty. Of course, a single estimate is
unlikely to be precisely accurate, but the estimates can still
be helpful over a range of different possibilities, and the
nomogram allows us to test the different levels at which
our estimates would change what we do. A helpful
discipline is to decide, in advance, what level of
probability would represent our threshold for making, or
not making, a particular management decision. So in this
case, we might have pushed for further investigation of
this man's back, perhaps by magnetic resonance imaging if
the probability of cancer was above 5%, but might have
been happy to wait and see if it were below this. In this
case, we can see that with pretest probabilities anywhere
above about 5%, the post-test probability of disease, in the
presence of a negative X-ray, would be higher than our
threshold for action. So, a completely precise estimate of
pretest probability is not necessary – just a reasonable
estimate, which we of course make intuitively every
day.

The evidence-based medicine (EBM) approach: was it worth it?

Experienced doctors who hear about this problem often say that they would not have placed as much value on the negative X-ray as we did. This may or may not be true. However, despite our being reasonably experienced clinicians, we had allowed ourselves, in the presence of a confusing picture, to place undue reliance on this particular test. For us, it was helpful both for this specific problem, and more generally for our approach to diagnostic tests, to work through this problem. As primary care doctors, it was heartening that, in the process, we reaffirmed the prime importance of clinical findings.

This problem may be less interesting to others who have not faced this particular scenario, or felt they already knew what value to place on X-rays in back pain. The message, for those interested in EBM, must surely be to spend your time and energy in tackling questions that are important to you. These may be critical incidents in your practice (as in our case), and/or problems that are so common and important (for example, when to treat elevated cholesterol levels with drugs) that the knowledge found can be applied again to patients with similar problems. Another important issue raised by this example is that evidence does not have to be perfect to be useful. The paper which we used as our source of evidence was not directed to answering our particular question. Indeed, the main conclusions of the paper are directed towards defining an algorithm to limit X-ray and other investigations to patients at higher risk of cancer through clinical findings. The authors were not setting out to determine what to do with patients with cancer who came up with negative findings on simple tests. Nevertheless, we were able to gather information from the study to help us answer just this question — and subsequently to change our clinical practice.

References

Deyo R A, Diehl A K 1988 Cancer as a cause of back pain: frequency, clinical presentation, and diagnostic strategies. Journal of General Internal Medicine 3: 230–238

Deyo R A, Rainville J, Kent D L 1992 What can the history and physical examination tell us about low back pain? Journal of the American Medical Association 268: 760–765

Fagan T J 1975 Letter: Nomogram for Bayes theorem. New England Journal of Medicine 293: 257

Jaeschke R, Guyatt G, Sackett D L 1994a Users' guides to the medical literature. III How to use an article about a diagnostic test. A Are the results of the study valid? Journal of the American Medical Association 271: 389–391

Jaeschke R, Guyatt G, Sackett D L 1994b Users' guides to the medical literature. III How to use an article about a diagnostic test. B What are the results and will they help me in caring for my patients? Journal of the American Medical Association 271: 703–707

McKibbon K A, Walker-Dilks C J 1994 Beyond ACP Journal Club: How to harness Medline for diagnostic problems. ACP Journal Club 121: A10–A12

Richardson W S, Wilson M C, Nishikawa J, Hayward R S 1995 The well-built clinical question: a key to evidence-based decisions (editorial). ACP Journal Club 123: A12–A13

© *Journal of General Internal Medicine* 1988; **3**: 230–238

Cancer as a Cause of Back Pain:
Frequency, Clinical Presentation, and Diagnostic Strategies

Richard A. Deyo, MD, MPH, Andrew K. Diehl, MD, MSc

Back pain is very common. Rarely, it may be the first manifestation of cancer. Although many advocate selective use of laboratory and x-ray tests for back pain patients, the early detection of cancer may be an important reason to obtain such tests. To develop a diagnostic approach that would identify malignancies while remaining parsimonious, the authors evaluated 1,975 walk-in patients with a chief complaint of back pain. Thirteen patients (0.66%) proved to have underlying cancer. Findings significantly associated with underlying cancer (p < 0.05) were: age ≥ 50 years, previous history of cancer, duration of pain > 1 month, failure to improve with conservative therapy, elevated erythrocyte sedimentation rate (ESR), and anemia. Combining historical features and ESR results led to an algorithm that would have limited x-ray utilization to just 22% of subjects while recommending an x-ray for every cancer patient.

It would further suggest which patients with negative x-ray findings require further work-up. Key words: cancer; back pain; clinical strategies; x-ray utilization. J GEN INTERN MED 1988; 3: 230–238.

Received from the Division of General Internal Medicine, Department of Medicine, The University of Texas Health Science Center at San Antonio, San Antonio, Texas, and the Seattle Veterans Administration Medical Center, Seattle, Washington.

Supported in part by a grant from the Robert Wood Jonnson Foundation, Princeton, New Jersey, and by the Northwest Health Services Research and Development Field Program, Seattle V.A. Medical Center.

The opinions, conclusions and proposals in the text are those of the authors, and do not necessarily represent the views of the Robert Wood Johnson Foundation.

Presented in part at the tenth annual meeting of the Society for Research and Education in Primary Care Internal Medicine, San Diego. April 30, 1987.

Address correspondence and reprint requests to Dr. Deyo: Health Services Research and Development, Seattle V.A. Medical Center, 1660 South Columbian Way, Seattle. WA 98108.

Back pain is the second leading symptom prompting patients to visit the doctor.[1] Among outpatients, it is the symptom most often associated with x-ray use.[2] Although serious underlying disease is rare in patients who have back complaints, the detection of malignancy or infection is a major goal of the diagnostic evaluation.[3] Metastatic cancer, the most common of these serious underlying diseases,[4] may manifest few other signs of its presence.

Although cancer-related back pain (usually due to spinal metastases) suggests that any underlying tumor is already advanced, there is probably therapeutic value in prompt diagnosis. Because cancer mandates specific therapy, we may presume that prompt detection will lead to earlier relief of suffering. Among patients destined to develop spinal cord compression, back pain almost always precedes neurologic deficits,[5] and timely detection of epidural cord compression may prevent substantial disability.

While cancers are a heterogeneous group of disorders, it is reasonable to consider them together in evaluating low back pain. For patients with this chief complaint, various forms of cancer have resulted in similar clinical presentations. The diagnostic methods for detecting spinal metastases (e.g., x-ray, bone scan), the complications of spinal

Continued →

metastases, and the therapeutic options (steroids, radiation, surgery) are similar regardless of the primary site. Finally, since all forms of cancer are probably the underlying cause of the pain in less than 1% of patients with back pain,[4] the initial clinical task is to 'rule in' or 'rule out' malignancy, rather than to comprehensively assess every organ from which metastases might arise.

However, there is persistent controversy regarding the proper initial evaluation of patients with back pain. Lumbar spine films are frequently obtained, but have a low yield, may be misleading, and result in large aggregate costs.[6] Some observers suggest that selective use of diagnostic tests (especially radiography) could reduce costs without missing serious underlying diseases.[6–9] Thus, we sought criteria by which certain patients could be spared x-ray examinations, while remaining assured that underlying malignancies would not go undiagnosed.

For x-ray ordering criteria, we considered historical, physical, and laboratory data that have been found to be associated with underlying cancer.[9–13] We had previously tested the screening value of several items of clinical data among early enrollees in this study (n = 621).[13] Four patients had cancer, all of whom had clinical findings to suggest the need for x-rays. We hoped to confirm the success of these clinical findings as screening tools and to determine whether inexpensive laboratory tests could improve the specificity of the clinical evaluation.

We therefore prospectively collected data in a primary care setting from a large series of patients complaining of back pain. We sought to estimate the prevalence of cancer as an underlying cause of back pain; to observe how frequently it is clinically unsuspected; to determine which items of the history and physical examination are most useful in its detection; and to examine the performances of several potential 'screening' tests for cancer among patients with low back pain. We

hoped the resulting data would suggest an economical algorithm for distinguishing those patients who had underlying cancers from the large majority with mechanical back pain.

Methods

Patients and data collection

All patients sought treatment between March 1982 and September 1984 in the walk-in clinic of a public hospital. This clinic is a source of primary care for indigent persons in a county of approximately one million population. Virtually all patients are self-referred. In each case, back pain was part of the chief complaint. Patients were examined by house-staff physicians from the Departments of Medicine, Family Practice, and Surgery. A standard coding form, adapted from previous studies of back pain,[9,14] was used to record 65 items of history and physical examination at the index visit. A listing of study subjects was maintained so that the same patient was not entered twice if two or more visits were made.

Laboratory and radiographic testing were performed at the discretion of the examining physician. On the basis of prior literature, it was recommended to houseofficers that an erythrocyte sedimentation rate (ESR) and a complete blood count (CBC) be obtained for most patients, but this was not an enforced policy. A strictly uniform testing approach was not implemented because 1) we did not feel there was sufficient basis in the literature for including or excluding certain tests for all patients as a routine procedure, 2) some patients had relative contraindications to x-ray testing (e.g., women without contraception, persons recently x-rayed), and 3) we could not provide uniform x-ray and laboratory testing as research procedures for a large number of patients. Because all

Continued →

patients did not receive all tests, certain analyses are limited to subsets of patients for whom particular tests were obtained.

Test results were recorded after the visit by searching computerized laboratory and radiology files. Because tests might have been done shortly before or after the index visit, we accepted ESR and CBC results obtained within 30 days of the index visit. All tests were done in the routine clinical laboratory, using the Westergren method for ESR determination.

We accepted x-ray results obtained within six months of the index visit (before or after), although more than 30% of x-rays were done within a week of the index visit. Among the 13 patients who had underlying cancers, two did not have spinal x-rays, six had x-rays within a week of the index visit, and five obtained x-rays five weeks to three months after the index visit. Of the five whose x-rays were delayed, two had no systemic sign or symptom at the index visit, and three had known cancer diagnoses (but metastasis was initially considered unlikely). The radiologist's official report was used for all x-ray results. Radiologists had available clinical data entered on the x-ray request form, which could have biased interpretation. However, cancer was not suspected for over half the patients who had it, making it unlikely that biasing information was provided in these cases. Our method of identifying cancer patients was independent of x-ray findings (see below).

Identification of underlying cancer

To identify patients who proved to have an underlying malignancy, we searched for each name in the institutional tumor registry at least six months after the index visit. We reasoned that this was sufficient time for occult metastatic cancer to become apparent and to be diagnosed. The registry included every patient with a histologic diagnosis of cancer made in our hospital system, regardless of the actual site of care. While this method might fail to identify cancer patients who sought care elsewhere, it is likely that most patients sought follow-up for a particular illness at the same facility. Among a subset of study subjects who participated in a clinical trial, 75% described our facility as their only source of care. This clinic population is largely indigent, with many patients having unstable housing and / or no telephone, so we believed this method of follow-up would be more complete than attempted telephone contact.

When a patient was identified in the tumour registry we made note of the date of cancer diagnosis, tumor type, and stage. On the basis of chronology, tumor location, stage, and imaging procedures, a judgment was made regarding the relationship between the tumor and back symptoms. For example, basal cell carcinomas of the skin and non-invasive cancers of the uterine cervix (often diagnosed and treated years before the index visit) were judged unrelated to back pain when there was no other clinical evidence of recurrence.

Analysis

We analyzed those clinical findings from the standard coding form that others have suggested are associated with malignancy.[9-13] Sensitivities and specificities of various findings for the diagnosis of cancer were calculated in the usual manner.[15] For each finding, we then calculated the 'likelihood ratio,' defined as the prevalence of a given finding in patients with underlying cancer divided by the prevalence of the finding in patients without cancer. This is equivalent to test sensitivity divided by 1 – specificity. Likelihood ratios greater than one indicate that the finding is more common in patients with cancer than in those without.[15] For

Continued →

continuous laboratory data (ESR, hematocrit, white blood cell count), receiver operating characteristic (ROC) curves were also developed. These curves plot sensitivity (true-positive rate) versus 1 – specificity (false-positive rate) for each of several cutoff points used to define a 'positive' test. The areas under these curves indicate the abilities of the tests to discriminate patients with cancer from those without.[15]

Finally, we selected those findings with the highest likelihood ratios to develop a rudimentary algorithm for diagnostic evaluation, seeking an approach which would have 100% sensitivity for cancer, but minimize laboratory or x-ray use. Discriminant analysis was used to determine which clinical and laboratory findings had the best independent abilities to distinguish between patients with and without cancer. In developing an algorithm, however, we used variables not in the discriminant model to achieve 100% sensitivity. The proportions of patients with cancer in clinically defined subgroups were estimated, and 95% confidence intervals were calculated.[16,17]

Results

Study population

There were 1,975 patients, ranging in age from 15 to 86 years (mean, 39.5 years, SD = 15.4). Sixty-two per cent were women. Many were seeking medical care for back pain for the first time (54%), and 76% had had pain for less than three months. Only 3% had a history of prior back surgery. Maximal pain was in the low back for 84% and in the upper back for 16% (neck pain was excluded). In this clinic, most patients are indigent and poorly educated, and a majority are Mexican-American, but specific data on income, education, and ethnicity were not collected for the entire sample. For a subset of 833 subjects who had x-rays of the lumbar spine,

we determined ethnicity from the hospital's computerized data file. In this subset, 73.6% were Mexican-American, 13.5% were white (non-Hispanic), and 12.9% were black.

Patients with cancer

Of the 1,975 study subjects, 38 were found in the tumor registry. However, only 13 had tumors that were probable causes of back pain at the index visit. Of the 25 whose cancers were judged unrelated to current back symptoms, 11 had cervical cancers (diagnosed an average of eight years previously); four had endometrial cancers (diagnosed an average of six years earlier); two had basal cell carcinomas on the face; two had ovarian cancers; two had breast cancers; and one each had a diagnosis of parotid mucoepidermoid cancer, leiomyosarcoma of the duodenum, melanoma of a finger, and lung cancer. In all but two cases, the diagnosis had been made before the index visit, usually many years previously. In each case there was no evidence of recurrence for at least six months after the index visit. The two patients whose cancers were diagnosed after the index visit had breast cancer and lung cancer, discovered eight months and one month after the index visit, respectively. In each case, bone scans performed after the diagnosis was made were negative, x-rays of the spine showed degenerative changes, and other evidence of metastases was absent (except for a positive axillary node in the patient with breast cancer).

Thus, underlying cancer as a cause of back pain was found in only 0.66% (13/1,975) of patients in this primary care practice. Table 1 shows demographic and clinical features of these 13 patients. Ten were more than 50 years old, four had a known cancer diagnosis at the time of the index visit, and in only six

Continued →

Table 1 Clinical and Demographic Features of 13 Patients with Cancer as a Cause of Back Pain

	Age (Years), Sex	Tumor Diagnosis	Cancer Known Prior to Back Symptoms	Signs or Symptoms of Systemic illness	Cancer Considered at Index Visit?	HCT (%)	ESR (mm/hr)	Spine X-ray Results
Patient 1	26.F	Lymphoma	No	Failure to improve with conservative therapy	No	40.0	29	Normal
Patient 2	62.M	Adenocarcinoma, unknown primary	No	None	No	38.0	53	Lytic lesions
Patient 3	52.M	Prostatic cancer	No	None	No	29.8*	45*	Blastic lesions
Patient 4	56.F	Retroperitoneal liposarcoma	No	Weight loss	No	31.1	133	Spondylolisthesis
Patient 5	51.M	Squamous carcinoma, lung	No	Weight loss	Yes	43.9*	Not done	Compression fractures
Patient 6	57.F	Renal cell carcinoma	No	Gross hematuria	No	40.8	Not done	Not done
Patient 7	65.F	Multiple myeloma	No	None	No	29.2	58	Compression fractures
Patient 8	36.F	Mucinous adenocarcinoma (?gallbladder)	No	Failure to improve with conservative therapy: abdominal pain	No	43.0	20	Not done
Patient 9	55.F	Lymphoma	No	Lymphadenopathy	Yes	40.8	17	Lytic lesions, compression fractures
Patient 10	34.F	Breast cancer	Yes	None	Yes	36.7	63	Blastic lesions
Patient 11	71.M	Squamous carcinoma, lung	Yes	Moderate weight loss: 9 pounds/3 mo	Yes	37.3	125	Osteopenia, degenerative joint disease
Patient 12	73.M	Prostatic cancer	Yes	None	Yes	39.2	Not done	Lytic and blastic lesions, compression fractures
Patient 13	51.F	Breast cancer	Yes	None	Yes	48.8	6	Lytic and blastic lesions

*Tests done more than one month after the index visit

Table 2 Clinical Findings among Patients with and Without Cancer as a Cause of Back Pain

	Prevalence in Patients with Underlying Cancer. i.e. Sensitivity (n^*)	Prevalence in Patients Without Cancer, i.e. 1 – Specificity (n^*)	Likelihood Ratio	Significance of Difference
History				
Age ≥ 50 years	0.77 (13)	0.29 (1.939)	2.7	p = 0.0005
Unexplained weight loss†	0.15 (13)	0.06 (1.938)	2.7	NS†
Previous history of cancer	0.31 (13)	0.02 (1.936)	14.7	p < 0.001
Sought medical care during past month, not improving	0.31 (13)	0.10 (1.962)	3.0	p = 0.05
Tried bedrest, but no relief	1.00 (4)	0.54 (939)	1.8	NS
Insidious onset	0.61 (13)	0.58 (1.935)	1.1	NS
Duration of this episode > 1 month	0.50 (12)	0.19 (1.890)	2.6	p = 0.02
Recent back injury (included lifting, fall, blow)	0 (13)	0.18 (1.952)	0	NS
Thoracic pain (vs. lumbar)	0.17 (12)	0.16 (1.920)	1.1	NS
Physical findings				
Appears to be in severe pain	0.23 (13)	0.15 (1.869)	1.6	NS
Muscle spasm	0.15 (13)	0.34 (1.858)	0.5	NS
Spine tenderness	0.15 (13)	0.40 (1.850)	0.4	NS
Neuromotor deficit	0 (12)	0.09 (1.774)	0	NS
Fever (temperature ≥ 100°F)	0 (13)	0.02 (1.946)	0	NS

*Exact numbers vary due to missing data or responses contingent on some prior action.
†Unexplained weight loss (by history) of more than 10 pounds in six months.
‡NS = not significant. p > 0.1.

cases was malignancy explicitly considered by the examining physician.

Among the nine patients with no prior cancer history, there were often delays from the index visit to the time of cancer diagnosis. The mean was 51 days, with three patients having delays of approximately three months.

Clinical findings in patients with and without cancer

Table 2 compares the prevalences of certain clinical findings among the 13 cancer patients and the roughly 1,900 patients without cancer. Findings that were significantly more common in patients with cancer included age of 50 years or more; having sought medical care during the past month (without relief); duration of pain longer than one month; and a prior history of cancer. While a third of patients who had underlying cancers had a known prior malignancy, only 2% of patients without underlying cancer had this history. This resulted in the highest likelihood ratio (14.7) for any historical or physical examination item. Although the associations were not statistically significant, unexplained weight loss and the absence of recent back injury were also associated with cancer, the former having a likelihood ratio greater than 2.0. Failure of bed rest to relieve the pain was uniform among the cancer patients who reported trying this treatment, but over half

Continued →

the non-cancer patients also reported failure of bedrest to relieve the pain.

Table 2 also provides data for physical examination findings. None of the physical signs were significantly associated with underlying cancer. Physicians judged patients to be in severe pain somewhat more frequently in the cancer group, but the likelihood ratio was only 1.6. Muscle spasm and spine tenderness were actually somewhat less common in patients with cancer. At the index visit, none of the cancer patients had neuromotor deficits, although at least two developed paraparesis later in the course of the disease. Thus, neurologic deficit appeared to be a late finding among the cancer patients. Neuromotor deficits were also infrequent (9%) among the non-cancer patients. Both patients who had prostatic cancer had rectal examinations performed at the index visit, but the results were said to be normal. Stool testing for occult blood (a single test) was performed for nine of the 13 cancer patients and was negative for all of them.

Laboratory findings

Since laboratory tests were not ordered uniformly, there were fewer cases available for assessing their performance. While selection of patients for laboratory testing was probably biased by clinical judgment, likelihood ratios have the desirable property of being quite stable in the face of changes in disease prevalence.[15]

We compared clinical and demographic features of those receiving and not receiving an ESR, a CBC, and a spinal x-ray to determine how the tested subgroups differed from the remaining patients. The patients who received an ESR were older than those who did not (40.8 years vs. 38.1 years), and had somewhat greater spinal flexibility. However, the two groups did not differ significantly with regard to sex, spinal

tenderness, weight loss, history of cancer, neurologic deficits, failure of previous therapy, duration of pain, or number of prior episodes of pain. Those receiving a CBC differed from those who did not in having higher proportions with spinal tenderness (44.8% vs. 37.3%) and fever (3.0% vs. 1.2%), and also in having slightly better spinal flexion. Those who received x-rays differed from those who did not in sex distribution (40.6% men vs. 35.7%) and in mean age (44 vs. 36 years). Patients who received x-rays were more often judged to have severe pain, muscle spasm, spinal tenderness, or neurologic deficits, had more often failed earlier therapy, and had slightly worse spinal flexion and straight-leg raising.

Table 3 shows the performances of the ESR, hematocrit (HCT), white blood cell count (WBC), and x-ray findings as 'screening tests' for cancer in patients with back pain. None of the tests was extremely sensitive, but the likelihood ratios for certain test results were substantially higher than those for history and physical findings.

The ESR was the most sensitive blood test, and its specificity exceeded those of the HCT and WBC at comparable levels of sensitivity. This is shown in Figure 1, which illustrates ROC curves for the ESR, HCT, and WBC. The ESR curve enclosed the largest area, and thus best distinguished patients with cancer from those without. The mean ESR for patients with underlying cancers was 56 mm/hr, as opposed to a mean of 16 mm/hr for patients without underlying cancer. The use of age- and sex-specific norms for the ESR[18] did not improve the likelihood ratio over an arbitrary cut-off of 20 mm/hour.

Any degree of anemia was a moderately useful discriminator between patients with and without cancer. More severe anemia (HCT < 30%) was associated with a greater likelihood ratio, but was present in only one

Continued →

Table 3 Laboratory Findings among Patients With and Without Cancer as a Cause of Back Pain

	Prevalence of Test Result in Patients with Underlying Cancer. i.e. Sensitivity (n^*)	Prevalence of Test Result in Patients Without Cancer. i.e. 1 – Specificity (n^*)	Likelihood Ratio	Significance of Difference
Erythrocyte sedimentation rate				
≥ 20 mm/hr	0.78 (9)	0.33 (999)	2.4	p = 0.01
≥ 50 mm/hr	0.56 (9)	0.03 (999)	19.2	p < 0.0001
≥ 100 mm/hr	0.22 (9)	0.004 (999)	55.5	p < 0.0001
Anemia[†]	0.54 (11)	0.14 (1.089)	4.0	p = 0.0006
Hematocrit < 30%	0.09 (11)	0.006 (1.089)	15.2	p = 0.13
WBC ≥ 12.000/cu mm	0.22 (9)	0.06 (528)	3.5	p = 0.21
X-ray				
Lytic or blastic lesion	0.60 (10)	0.005 (823)	120.0	p < 0.0001
Compression fracture	0.20 (10)	0.043 (823)	4.6	p = 0.10
Either compression fracture or lytic/blastic lesion	0.70 (10)	0.017 (823)	14.9	p < 0.0001

*Number of subjects varies because the test was not performed in all patients.
†Anemia was defined as a hematocrit less than 40% for men and less than 38% for women, the current standards in our clinical laboratory.

cancer patient, for a sensitivity of 9%. An elevated WBC (≥ 12,000/cu mm) was less useful as a diagnostic test, and altering the 'cut-off' value did not improve its performance. The ROC curve for WBC in Figure 1 falls almost on the diagonal line, indicating no ability to discriminate cancer patients from non-cancer patients.

As expected, the x-ray finding of lytic or blastic lesions was an excellent discriminator between patients with and without underlying cancer, though some false negatives and rare false positives did occur. Two cancer patients had compression fractures without lytic or blastic lesions. It seems likely that these were truly pathologic fractures, since they occurred in a patient with multiple myeloma, and in the thoracic spine of a patient with lung cancer. Since compression fractures were relatively common among patients without cancer, the discriminatory value of this finding was much less than that of lytic or blastic lesions. The greatest sensitivity for x-ray (70%)

resulted by counting either compression fractures or lytic/blastic lesions as positive findings, with a corresponding specificity of 95%.

Multivariate analysis

We used stepwise discriminant analysis to determine which of the findings in Tables 2 and 3 (other than x-ray results) had the greatest independent ability to distinguish between patients with and without underlying cancer. Such a discriminant rule might help to identify the small number of subjects with a sufficiently high probability of cancer that x-rays should be performed, while excluding from radiography those subjects with a low probability of cancer. This analysis was first performed using patients with complete clinical data who also received an ESR ($n = 929$). The only findings that entered the discriminant model were a

Continued →

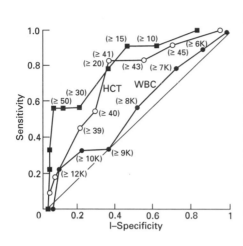

Fig. 1
Receiver operating characteristic (ROC) curves for the erythrocyte sedimentation rate (ESR), hematocrit (HCT), and white blood cell count (WBC) as tests for detecting cancer among patients with low back pain. Each point on the curves represents test performance using a particular 'cut-off' value to define a positive test. These 'cut-offs' are indicated in parentheses beside most data points. The curve enclosing the largest area (ESR) has the best ability to discriminate patients with underlying cancer from those without. The diagonal line represents a test with no ability to discriminate (the false-positive rate equals the true-positive rate for any test result).

history of prior cancer and the ESR result (both p < 0.0001). In an analysis including CBC results (*n* = 408 cases with complete data), neither the WBC nor the HCT entered the stepwise analysis. In the analysis including ESR as the only laboratory test, 97% of patients were correctly classified by the discriminant rule, using the actual prevalence of cancer in the study sample as the prior probability. While a history of cancer and the ESR alone might be efficient at classifying patients, the discriminant rule misclassified six cancer patients as non-cancer patients. Thus, we sought a broader group of findings that would be more sensitive for early evaluation, even at the expense of specificity. Such a rule might

insure that all patients with cancer received x-rays, while still excluding a substantial number of subjects for whom cancer was extremely unlikely.

Diagnostic strategies

From the data in Table 2, we selected the clinical findings with the highest likelihood ratios for cancer. In this study, every patient with cancer had at least one of the four clinical findings with the highest likelihood ratios: age greater than 50 years, history of cancer, unexplained weight loss, or failure to improve with conservative therapy. Thus, if further diagnostic tests had been limited only to patients with these clinical findings, no patient who had cancer would have been missed. This strategy alone would result in substantial savings over uniform radiography and laboratory testing for all patients with low back pain.

A more economical approach would be possible if patients were divided into three subgroups, based on clinical findings. 'High-risk' patients are those with a prior history of cancer. In our study, 9% of such patients proved to have cancer causing their back pain (4/45). For these, an immediate ESR and x-ray would be warranted, and a positive result on either would mandate further work-up. 'Low-risk' patients are those under age 50 with no history of cancer, no weight loss or other sign of systemic illness, and no history of failure to improve with conservative therapy. In our study, there were no cancers among 1,170 such patients (upper 95% CI = 0.3%). For these, a strategy of no laboratory or x-ray tests might be appropriate unless an indication arose during follow-up (e.g., failure to improve).

An 'intermediate-risk' group includes patients over age 50, those with a failure of conservative therapy, and those with

Continued →

unexplained weight losses or other signs of systemic illness (lymphadenopathy and hematuric in our study). In this group, 1.2% of subjects had cancer (95% CI = 0.4%, 2.0%). For the group, the ESR may be particularly useful in raising or lowering the suspicion of cancer. Based on the proportion of abnormal test results among subjects who received an ESR, we can estimate that 369 subjects had an ESR less than 20 mm/hr and only one of the clinical findings. No cancers were identified among such patients (upper 95% CI = 0.8%). On the other hand, for subjects with an ESR ≥ 20 mm/hr or with two or more clinical findings (e.g., age > years plus weight loss) nine of 391 subjects proved to have cancers (2.3%, with 95% CI = 0.8%, 3.8%). For these patients, prompt spinal radiography may be appropriate, although some who proved to have cancers had normal x-rays. Thus, persons who had elevated ESRs but normal x-rays would require close follow-up and/or additional diagnostic test. No patient in our study who had underlying cancer had both a normal x-ray and an ESR < 20 mm/hr (among those who had the tests done), so that further testing among such patients would have a very low yield. Figure 2 presents a simple algorithm based on these considerations, and indicates the consequences among our study subjects. This algorithm would have limited x-ray use to just 22% of subjects and would have recommended an x-ray for every cancer patient.

Discussion

This study supports several conclusions concerning the detection of cancer in patients presenting with back pain. First, the prevalence of underlying cancers among back pain patients in an unselected primary care population is low: approximately seven cases per 1,000 patients. Second, patients with underlying malignancies often have few suggestive signs, and the diagnosis is often initially overlooked. Nonetheless, there are features of the history that should raise the suspicion of cancer and prompt a directed laboratory and radiograph evaluation. Third, the ESR is a useful screening tool when applied selectively. Along with suggestive historical findings, an elevated ESR should prompt radiography. Fourth, in the face of suggestive historical findings and an elevated ESR, a 'negative' x-ray of the spine should be interpreted with caution. Clinical follow-up and additional diagnostic tests may be indicated in this situation. And fifth, using the history and ESR, it is possible to select groups of low-risk patients who do not need early radiography, resulting in substantial cost savings.

Because 90% of patients who have mechanical pain improve within a month,[19] longitudinal observation is an important diagnostic tool. This is reflected in our algorithm, which recommends no testing for the lowest-risk subjects (a majority of this sample) unless indications subsequently arise. It is also reflected in the use of 'failure of conservative therapy' as an indication for testing. In subjects with previous cancers, age over 50, or unexplained weight losses, the prior probability of cancer is sufficiently high (1–9%) that some immediate diagnostic testing appears warranted, assuming that earlier diagnosis leads to earlier relief of suffering. Costs of radiography per day of suffering averted appear reasonable for this range of probabilities ($43 to $558 per day, even without the greater selectivity that the ESR may permit).[4] In our study, not every subject had received a trial of conservative therapy at the index visit. Ideally, such follow-up data would have been available to construct an algorithm. However, the natural history of back pain is such that uniform return visits may be unnecessary, and rules for decision-making at a single visit may be important.

Continued →

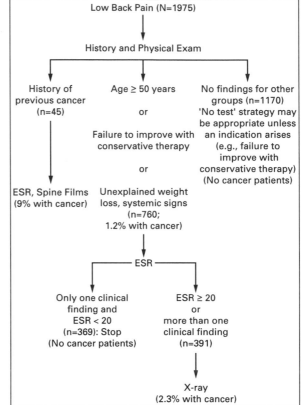

Fig. 2
One possible algorithm for detecting underlying cancer in patients with low back pain. The number of patients in our study who would fall into each subgroup is shown, along with the percentage who proved to have cancer. In some cases, subgroup sizes are estimates, based on the proportions of abnormal results and clinical findings among the subset of patients (*n* = 1.008) who actually had an erythrocyte sedimentation rate (ESR) performed. 'Systemic signs' refers to findings that would mandate investigation on their own: lymphadenopathy and hematuria were examples in our study.

The indications for radiography in Figure 2 are not the only ones to be considered in managing a patient with back pain. Radiography would also be indicated for patients with clinical findings that suggest underlying infection, fracture, or inflammatory spondylitis. Fortunately, the ESR is useful for detecting infectious and inflammatory diseases as well as cancer,[6] so only minor modifications of the algorithm may be necessary to broaden its diagnostic scope.

This study is consonant with earlier research in several respects. Bone scintigraphy (to detect cancer or osteomyelitis) was reported to be unhelpful in the management of patients who had normal radiographs and laboratory findings.[11] Fernbach and colleagues reported that 17 of 18 patients with cancers as a cause of back pain were over age 50, and the ESR was abnormal for 94%.[12] As in other series, the primary sites most often associated with spinal metastases in our study were breast, lung, and prostate.[20]

Nonetheless, some limitations of this study should be noted. First, with only 13 cancer patients, the results of our study should be generalized cautiously. Second, we could not ensure that all patients presenting to the

Continued →

walk-in clinic on nights or weekends would be included. We cannot precisely quantify the number of individuals who were excluded, but based on administrative records, we believe that two-thirds of all back pain patients presenting during the study period were included. Third, not all patients received every diagnostic test, and those who received tests were in some respects systematically different from the remainder. To the extent that 'sicker' patients were more likely to have tests done, our estimates of abnormal results among non-cancer patients may be inflated. Fourth, we cannot be certain that ascertainment of cancer cases was complete. If patients sought care elsewhere after the index visit, they might not appear in our tumor registry. We believe this is a small risk, since most patients in this walk-in clinic describe our institution as their only source of care. Since most were indigent, it also seems likely that they would come to our public hospital for expensive illnesses (such as cancer). Fifth, because only 13 subjects had cancer, the complexity of a multivariate statistical model for our data set was limited to just one or two predictive variables. Rather than seeking the best statistical classification rate, however, we have sought a highly sensitive rule even at the expense of recommending a number of negative work-ups. The intent was to minimize serious errors in patient care.

Finally, our results need to be validated in a separate group of patients. In part, we have tested previous hypotheses about the value of certain clinical or laboratory data in detecting underlying cancer. While the results are concordant with earlier work,[9-13] the algorithm should be validated independently to assess its generalizability. The rarity of cancer as a cause of back pain necessitates large studies for this purpose. Future studies may benefit from a policy accounting for previous x-rays, potentially allowing even more selective radiography.

Our data support the safety and value of selective x-ray use in the evaluation of patients with back pain. Application of such selective criteria holds the promise of substantially reducing costs of care without a decrement in quality. Judicious use of the ESR may allow even more selective x-ray use than that proposed[13] on the basis of history alone.

Margaret Moya, Helen Provot, and Nancy Sugarek provided expert technical assistance. Richard L. Bauer, MD, and Daniel Kent, MD, provided helpful reviews of an earlier version of the manuscript, Ms. Moya and Kathy Minotto assisted in preparing the manuscript. The cooperation of the housestaff of the Medical Center Hospital who completed clinical evaluations of the patients is greatly appreciated.

References

1. Cypress B K 1983 Characteristics of physician visits for back symptoms: a national perspective. Am J Public Health 73: 389–95
2. Kocn H, Gagnon R O 1979 Office visits involving x-rays. National Ambulatory Medical Care Survey: United States, 1977. Advance data from vital and health statistics. No. 53, DHEW Publication No. (PHS) 79–1250, pp 1–7
3. Hall F M, 1980 Back pain and the radiologist. Radiology 137: 861–3
4. Liang M, Komaroff A L 1982 Roentgenograms in primary care patients with acute low back pain: a cost-effectiveness analysis. Arch Intern Med 142: 108–12
5. Gilbert T C W, Kim J, Posner J B 1978 Epidural spinal cord compression from metastatic tumor: diagnosis and treatment. Ann Neurol 3: 40–51
6. Deyo R A 1986 The early diagnostic evaluation of low back pain. J Gen Intern Med 1: 328–38
7. Nachemson A L 1976 The lumbar spine: an orthopedic challenge. Spine 1: 59–71
8. Fries J F, Mitchell D M 1976 Joint pain or arthritis. JAMA 235: 199–204
9. Rockey P H, Tompkins R K, Wood R W, Wolcott B W 1978 The usefulness of x-ray examinations in the evaluation of patients with back pain. J Fam Pract 7: 455–65
10. MacNab I 1977 Backache, Baltimore: Williams and Wilkins. 131–2
11. Schutte H E, Park W M 1983 The diagnostic value of

Continued →

bone scintigraphy in patients with low back pain. Skeletal Radiol 10: 1–4

12. Fernbach J C, Langer F, Gross A E 1976 The significance of low back pain in older adults. Can Med Assoc J 115: 898–900

13. Deyo R A, Diehl A K 1986 Lumbar spine films in primary care: current use and effects of selective ordering criteria. J Gen Intern Med 1: 20–5

14. Greenfield S, Anderson H, Winickoff R N et al. 1975 Nurse-protocol management of low back pain. West J Med 123: 350–9

15. Sackett D L, Haynes R B Tugwell P 1985 Clinical epidemiology: a basic science for clinical medicine. Boston. Little, Brown. 59–138

16. Hanley J A, Lippman-Hand A 1983 If nothing goes wrong, is everything all right? Interpreting zero numerators. JAMA 249: 1743–5

17. Bulpitt C J 1987 Confidence intervals. Lancet i: 494–7

18. Miller A, Green M, Robinson D 1983 Simple rule for calculating normal erythrocyte sedimentation rate. Br Med J 286: 266

19. Dillane J B, Fry J, Katton G 1966 Acute back syndrome – a study from general practice. Br Med J 2: 82–4

20. Schaberg J, Gainor B J 1985 A profile of metastatic carcinoma of the spine. Spine 10: 19–20

CHAPTER 5

What is the likely outcome when patients present with psychological problems?
An approach to evidence from studies of prognosis

Leone Ridsdale

The clinical problem

Mrs Jones came in saying her husband wanted her to 'get something for PMT' There was a long history of marital disharmony and she was depressed. I asked if they had considered separating. She replied that this was impossible as her husband would not move out of the house and she would not move with the children into a flat. I wondered what was likely to happen to her in the long run, and what role the practice might have.

I came to my GP training fresh from working in an outpatient psychiatry clinic. At that time about a third of GP trainees, and a lower proportion of GPs and trainers, had done postgraduate training in psychiatry. We were frequently asked to bring 'problem patients' for discussion at our day-release course. Almost invariably, trainees would come with a thick wedge of notes and a long story, usually about a female patient with psychological problems. The diagnosis and treatment often remained unclear, but the individual trainee seemed to obtain some relief that other trainees and practices felt similarly burdened and impotent. It was unusual for us to look for anything more than a sharing of common experience, which helped us develop a sense of what it was like to cope outside the familiar territory of hospital medicine. I became fascinated with discovering the outcome of such patients.

In 1981 Jenkins, Mann and Belsey published two interesting reports of the 12 months outcome of 100 patients who presented with neurotic illness in two general practices. They suggested that social factors and symptom severity were significantly associated with outcome at one year, but that the GP's or the psychiatrist's diagnosis was not. I felt reassured that getting the diagnosis right was not all that important from the point of view of outcome. The importance of social factors supported some of the cherished beliefs that I acquired during my preparation for the Royal College of General Practitioners examinations.

A few years later I read and reviewed Dr John Fry's pioneering work in this area done 25 years previously in his own practice (Ridsdale 1985). Fry had set up an age/sex morbidity register and reported on the demographic characteristics and high attendance rate of patients with a neurotic illness. Three years later Wilkinson et al (1988) followed up on Fry's patients. They found that his patients with a psychological problem had an increased consulting rate over 20 years; some of this, they suggested, was due to (co-morbid) physical illness.

Fry's work was remarkable. Perhaps it stimulated researchers in psychiatry, more than any other specialty, to cross the boundaries and investigate symptoms in the community. Jenkins and Mann later followed up and reported on their general practice cohort after 11 years (Lloyd et al 1996). This paper addressed my questions about the likely long-term outcome for Mrs Jones so I decided to appraise it using Sackett et al's (1997) guidelines. The questions to be applied to a paper on prognosis are shown below.

Is this evidence about prognosis valid?

1. Was the defined representative sample of patients assembled at a common (usually early) point in the course of their disease?
2. Was patient follow-up sufficiently long and complete?
3. Were objective outcome criteria applied in a 'blind' fashion?
4. If subgroups with different prognoses are identified:
   — was there adjustment for important prognostic factors?
   — was there validation in an independent group of test set patients?

Is this evidence about prognosis important?

1. How likely are the outcomes over time?
2. How precise are the prognostic estimates?

1. Was the defined representative sample of patients assembled at a common (usually early) point in the course of their disease?

In their paper Lloyd et al (1996) reported that the sampling frame was selected to reproduce the range of patients reported in the 1974 national morbidity survey in general practice. The national morbidity survey had derived its data from all consultations in 60 practices with a total population of 300 000 patients in England and Wales for 1 year (Crombie & Fleming 1986). More details about the sample selection in Lloyd's study was provided in their original papers (Mann et al 1981, Jenkins et al 1981). Attending patients over 16 were asked to complete the 30-item General Health Questionnaire (GHQ) in the waiting room of the two surgeries on one day each week. Only those patients who agreed to do this were considered eligible for the study. Volunteers who had a positive score of 4 or more were eligible to enter the study. The research psychiatrist examined the notes and then questioned the general practitioner (GP). Only if the GP recognized a psychiatric disorder was the patient asked to join the study and undergo a psychiatric research interview. The patients who were not recognized by their GP or who refused to enter the study were not described.

It is difficult to know how much bias might be introduced by patients either not agreeing to fill in a questionnaire or attend a research interview, or by their GP failing to recognize an illness, and in what way the absence of these people might affect the outcome of the study. None the less, the investigators had clearly specified their criteria so that patients would be recruited who would be likely to have similar characteristics to other patients in the much larger general practice morbidity survey.

The second component of this question on critical appraisal asks whether patients were recruited at a common (usually early) point in the course of their illness. From the criteria specified by the investigators, it seems likely that the sample of patients were recruited at different points in the course of their disease. Some may have had an acute onset. However, it is likely that many of them had relapsing, remitting or chronic symptoms. If GPs were more likely to recognize psychological illness when it was relapsing/remitting or chronic, then this sample might be less likely to include patients, for example, with their first episode of neurotic illness, presenting perhaps initially with physical symptoms or in association with a physical illness (Freeling et al 1985, Tylee et al 1993). In other cohort studies such as one on fatigue, duration of symptoms on admission predicted good or poor outcome at follow-up (Ridsdale et al 1993), with longer duration of symptoms being associated with a worse outcome. It would have been useful therefore if information had been provided about the duration of the psychological symptoms when patients entered the study. None the less, the method of recruitment, which matched the sample recruited to the characteristics of a much larger sample drawn from general practice, makes it likely that GPs could infer from these attenders to their own patients in general practice.

2. Was patient follow-up sufficiently long and complete?

The interval before follow-up was impressively long at 11 years, and in view of this it was also impressive that 87 of the subjects were traced. Only 13 of the patients could not be traced after 11 years; an additional 19/87 had died, and causes of death were established, presumably for all these deaths. If all 13 drop-outs had died, the mortality rate would have risen to 32/100 (32%); but those who died were on average significantly older, whilst those who were lost to follow-up were significantly younger. If none of these lost to follow-up died, the mortality would have been 19%.

3. Were objective outcome criteria applied in a 'blind' fashion?

It seems likely that the idea of following the patients up 11 years later was not considered at the beginning of the study, so a plan for what criteria to use for measuring outcome was not prespecified. Some outcomes were objective and reproducible: for example, death. However, none of the deaths could be regarded as the outcome of psychological illness: for example, suicide. They occurred predominantly in older patients with an average age of 75, and were from common causes like cardiovascular disease, respiratory disease and malignancy.

Average annual consultation frequency derived from the GP records among this cohort was over 10 throughout the period. This was more than twice the average level found in the general practice morbidity survey (Crombie & Fleming 1986). Lloyd et al's (1996) finding is objective information, but one cannot be sure whether it is reproducible and accurate. This would depend on the extent to which the two practices kept their notes in a methodical, possibly tagged fashion, so that cards were not misplaced which might lead to under-recording of consultation frequency. It is possible that the consultation levels extracted from the notes could understate the frequency with which the patients actually consulted. If a comparison group of, say, 100 attenders with no psychological problem had been enlisted, or 100 non-consulters from the doctors' list, then a comparison might have been made between them.

Psychiatric outcome was measured by using the 12-item GHQ, by reference to the case notes, and by patient self-report. The GHQ has been shown to be a valid and reliable instrument with which to measure psychological distress in the community (Goldberg & Williams 1988). Jenkins et al (1988) have shown that general practitioners' classification of mental disorders is by no means reproducible or accurate, and it may be that the patient self-reports were more likely to provide accurate information.

Interestingly, there was no association found between initial assessment of social problems and psychiatric outcomes, as was found previously (Jenkins et al 1981). However, in order to measure this there had initially been a structured interview in which social stresses and supports had been recorded. This was converted into a questionnaire for follow-up purposes, but no description was provided about the reproducibility and accuracy of information derived in this way.

No research assistant or statistician is named either as a co-author or in the acknowledgements. It is not clear if Lloyd extracted data from the notes (which was unlikely to be blind) and analysed the data too.

4. If subgroups with different prognoses are identified, was there adjustment for important prognostic factors? Was there validation in an independent group of test set patients?

Multiple regression analysis was undertaken, with adjustment for age and sex. High initial GHQ score was strongly associated with high GHQ score at 11 years, chronic course of psychiatric illness, and high consultations, with and without adjustment for age and sex. The elevated standardized mortality ratio for this group, and their reasons for death, suggest that the cohort had a higher frequency of organic illness than other patients.

Mann et al (1981) reported that the psychiatrist classified physical illnesses, presumably from the records, according to whether they were acute, chronic, severe or painful. The extent to which this was an accurate or reproducible process is not clear. From the information provided it is evident that some of these patients had chronic physical illness, anteceding their recruitment into the study. These physical illnesses might also lead to psychological distress, frequent consulting and a higher death rate. When they adjusted for age, sex and chronic physical illness, the association between high attendance in primary care and chronic psychiatric course was reduced by more than one-half. This suggests that although there was a significant association between high attendance and a chronic psychological course, chronic physical illness may explain at least some of the excess attendance and chronic psychiatric symptoms. The interrelationship between physical and psychological illness is perhaps the most difficult aspect of work such as this.

At the time of follow-up the investigators knew that the relationship of characteristics at recruitment with outcomes would be described retrospectively. On the basis of their findings, inferences and new hypotheses might be drawn which could be tested on an independent group of patients. This might have also been possible by randomly selecting two subgroups from the total sample, finding associations in one group, and then testing them on another. However, given the relatively small number of patients (68) with full case notes and patient report data available, the sample size was too small to do this.

Is this evidence about prognosis important?

I believe that it is relevant and useful to know about the likely long-term outcomes when patients present with neurotic illness in general practice. From this study it is clear that these patients increased general practitioner workload quite substantially and this confirms the findings of Wilkinson et al (1988). When Lloyd et al (1996) followed up on this cohort of patients, those with a chronic psychiatric course were nearly 5 times as likely to consult more than 12 times per year during the follow-up period. The 95% confidence interval for the associated odds ratio is from 1.12 to 20.28, indicating a significantly raised consultation level for this group. (A short definition of confidence intervals and other statistical terms is provided in the glossary at the end of the book). High GHQ scores on entry were associated with high GHQ scores after 11 years, chronic psychiatric course and high consultation frequency. Of those who consulted with neurotic illness 52% had high symptom scores 11 years later. This may make some clinicians have a sense of heartsink, nihilism, challenge, or a wish that patients like this would register somewhere else, or that there was a fee-for-service remuneration that rewarded doctors for the increased workload.

In Lloyd et al's (1996) study the patients who presented with neurotic illness were more likely to die with a standardized mortality ratio of 173 (95% confidence interval, 164 to 200). The authors point out that the sample size was relatively small so the confidence intervals are quite wide in most of their prognostic estimates. From what has been stated previously, the increased mortality ratio may not be important, except as a reminder that physical illness is frequently accompanied by psychological distress.

The conclusion of the investigators is: 'These findings highlight the need for early identification and prompt and effective treatment of patients with neurotic disorders.'

Johnstone & Goldberg (1976) have suggested that the GHQ might be used as a screening tool in general practice, and if general practitioners acted on the results of high symptom scores, the duration and severity of psychological symptoms might be ameliorated. On the basis of a trial, Hollyman and colleagues (1988) suggested that amitriptyline taken in therapeutic doses significantly improved depressed patients' symptoms 4 weeks later. Marks (1985) and Ross & Scott (1985) have demonstrated that cognitive therapy can also benefit these patients.

During the 1990s a lot of attention has been focused on improving the diagnostic and therapeutic skills of general practitioners, particularly in the management of depression (Paykel & Priest 1992), and perhaps it is still too early to evaluate this programme. However, it may be difficult to demonstrate a health gain. When German et al (1987) used the GHQ as a screening tool by family doctors in the United States, they could not demonstrate the benefit found by

Johnstone and Goldberg (1976). Wilkinson et al (1988) examined the potential effect of new prescriptions of a psychotropic drug on consulting frequency among Dr Fry's patients, and could not show there was an offset effect of active treatment on general health care. A continuing problem is the known interaction between physical and psychological illness. There is also a relationship between social disadvantage, like threatened unemployment, depression and attendance at the doctor (Beale & Nethercott 1985). If unemployment increased as a trend, it might cancel out health gain derived, for example, through a 'successful' Defeat Depression campaign. Notwithstanding this complex social process, I believe Lloyd and his colleagues' paper contributes importantly to our understanding of the natural history of neurotic illness in general practice.

References

Beale N, Nethercott S 1985 Job loss and family morbidity: a study of a factory closure. Journal of the Royal College of General Practitioners 35: 510–514

Crombie D L, Fleming D M 1986 Comparison of second national morbidity study and general household survey 1970–71. Health Trends 18: 15–18

Freeling P, Rao B M, Paykel E S, Sireling L I, Burton R H 1985 Unrecognized depression in general practice. British Medical Journal 29: 1880–1883

German P S, Shapiro S, Skinner A E A, Von Korff M, Klein L E, Turner R W, Teitelbaum M L, Burke J, Burnes B J 1987 Detection and management of mental health problems of older patients by primary care providers. Journal of the American Medical Association 257: 489–493

Goldberg D, Williams P 1988 A user's guide to the general health questionnaire (GHQ). NFER-Nelson, Windsor

Hollyman J A, Freeling P, Paykel E S, Bhat A, Sedgwich P 1988 Double-blind placebo-controlled trial of amitriptyline among depressed patients in general practice. Journal of the Royal College of General Practitioners 38: 393–397

Jenkins R, Mann A H, Belsey E 1981 The background, design and use of a short interview to assess social stress and support in research and clinical settings. Social Science and Medicine 15: 195–203

Jenkins R, Smeeton N, Shepherd M 1988 Classification of mental disease in primary care. Psychological Medicine (Monograph suppl 12)

Johnstone A, Goldberg D 1976 Psychiatric screening in general practice: a controlled trial. Lancet i: 605–608

Lloyd K R, Jenkins R, Mann A 1996 Long term outcome of patients with neurotic illness in general practice. British Medical Journal 313: 26–28

Mann A H, Jenkins R, Belsey E 1981 The 12 month outcome of patients with neurotic disorder in general practice. Psychological Medicine 11: 535–550

Marks I 1985 Controlled trial of psychiatric nurse therapists in primary care. British Medical Journal 290: 1181–1184

Paykel E S, Priest R G on behalf of consensus participants 1992 Recognition and management of depression in general practice: consensus statement. British Medical Journal 305: 1198–1202

Ridsdale L 1985 Neurosis in general practice: 25 years on. Practitioner 229: 679–680

Ridsdale L, Evans A, Jerrett W, Mandalia S, Osler K, Vora H 1993 Patients with fatigue in general practice: a prospective study. British Medical Journal 307: 103–106

Ross M, Scott M 1985 An evaluation of the effectiveness of individual and group cognitive therapy in the treatment of depressed patients in an inner city health centre. Journal of the Royal College of General Practitioners 35: 239–242

Sackett D L, Richardson W S, Rosenberg W, Haynes R B 1997 Evidence-based medicine: how to practise and teach EBM. Churchill Livingstone, London

Tylee A, Freeling P, Kerry S 1993 Why do general practitioners recognize major depression in one woman patient yet miss it in another? British Journal of General Practice 43: 327–330

Wilkinson G, Smeeton N, Skuse D, Fry J 1988 Consultations for psychiatric illness by patients diagnosed and treated for psychiatric disorders by a general practitioner: 20 year follow-up study. British Medical Journal 297: 776–778

© British Medical Journal 1996; 313: 26–8

Long term outcome of patients with neurotic illness in general practice

Keith R Lloyd, Rachel Jenkins, Anthony Mann

Abstract

Objective—To determine the 11 year outcome of neurotic disorder in general practice.

Design—Cohort study over 11 years.

Setting—Two general practices in Warwickshire England.

Subjects—100 patients selected to be representative of those identified nationally by general practitioners as having neurotic disorders.

Main outcome measures—Mortality, morbidity, and use of health services.

Results—At 11 years 87 subjects were traced. The 11 year standardised mortality ratio was 173 (95% confidence interval 164 to 200). 47 were cases on the general health questionnaire, 32 had a relapsing or chronic psychiatric course, and 49 a relapsing or chronic physical course. Treatment for psychiatric illness was mainly drugs. The mean number of consultations per year was 10.8 (median 8.7). A persistent psychiatric diagnosis at one year follow up was associated with high attendance (> 12 visits a year for 11 years) at follow up after age, sex, and physical illness were adjusted for. Severity of psychiatric illness (general health questionnaire score) at outset predicted general health questionnaire score at 11 year follow up, course of psychiatric illness, and high consultation rate.

Conclusion—These data support the view that a neurotic illness can become chronic and is associated with raised mortality from all causes and high use of services. Such patients need effective intervention, particularly those with a more severe illness who do not recover within one year.

Key messages

- People attending primary care with neurotic disorders have high psychiatric morbidity and increased mortality from all causes
- In this study almost half had a chronic course over 11 years
- Chronic neurotic disorder is associated with high consultation regardless of physical illness
- Initial severity at diagnosis is the best predictor of long term outcome and consultation rate
- Practices need to develop systems to identify and manage effectively people with these common mental disorders.

Mental Health Research Unit, University of Exeter, Exeter EX2 5DW
Keith R Lloyd, *senior lecturer*
Institute of Psychiatry, De Crespigny Park, London SE5 8AF
Rachel Jenkins, *senior lecturer*
Anthony Mann,
professor of epidemiological psychiatry
Correspondence to:
Dr Lloyd, k.r.lloyd@exeter.ac.uk

Introduction

General practitioners exclusively manage 95% of all patients with psychiatric disorders.[1] Two thirds of these patients have non-psychotic syndromes of 'neurotic disorders,' with depressive and anxiety symptoms predominating. Many cases go undetected.[2] In a study of patients with neurotic disorder in general practice a quarter

Continued →

had unremitting psychiatric symptoms at one year follow up.[4] Poorer outcome was associated with severity of initial psychiatric symptoms, serious physical illness, and fewer social supports. Social, material, and personality factors are also important determinants of outcome.[3,5]

Apart from the persisting morbidity, neurotic illness has high economic costs.[6,7] One reason for this is the relation with attendance at general practice. Among women, high attendance is associated with psychiatric morbidity, younger age, lower socioeconomic group, and concomitant physical symptoms.[8] Older people are less likely to attend unless they also have physical conditions or come from higher socioeconomic groups. Ethnicity, personality, and somatisation also affect use of health services.[5,10–12]

Short term outcomes of neurotic disorder have been reported, but little is known about long term outcomes. We report the outcome after 11 years in a group of patients who took part in an earlier one year study.[4]

Subjects and methods

One year follow up

The original cohort of 72 women and 28 men was recruited from two Warwickshire general practices. The sampling frame was selected to reproduce the range of patients reported in the 1974 national morbidity survey in general practice. The cohort was thus representative for age, sex, and diagnosis. The method of the original study has been described.[4] Consecutive attenders were screened with the general health questionnaire.[13] Those who scored 4 or more entered the study if the general practitioner also reported a psychiatric diagnosis under the international classification of diseases (ICD9). Recruitment continued until 100 patients of appropriate age, sex, and diagnosis had been discovered to complete the

cells of the sampling frame. The diagnoses were anxiety or phobic neurosis (33); depressive neurosis (56); physical disorders of psychogenic origin or tension headache (3); insomnia (2), other conditions (6).

Subjects were interviewed with the clinical interview schedule,[14] the social stresses and support interview,[15] and the standardised assessment of personality.[16]

At one year follow up 93 patients were reinterviewed. Two had died, three refused second interviews, and two had moved away. Interval assessments of mental state were recorded by the general practitioner during follow up.

11 Year follow up

For the 11 year follow up we traced patients through the family health services authorities and approached them for a follow up assessment. They were sent a 12 item general health questionnaire and a semistructured schedule to collect retrospective follow up information about social circumstances and health from patients' perspectives. The schedule followed the items of the social stresses and support interview to allow comparison. The self reported data were also compared with general practitioners' records for the same period. Case notes were examined for consultation frequency, continuing psychiatric symptoms, physical illness, prescription of psychotropic drugs, and social events.

Analysis of data

We calculated the 11 year standardised mortality ratio for Warwickshire using data from the Office of Censuses and Population Surveys. Patient outcomes were classified by two methods. Firstly, we used the general health questionnaire to assess caseness

Continued →

(threshold score of 3) and total score according to the general health questionnaire method.[13]

Secondly, we used the pattern of the psychiatric disorder over the previous 11 years as shown in the case notes and the patients' reports. Classification of outcome was the same as in the one year follow up: well (the patient had no more psychiatric illness after the index episode); acute (the patient and the case notes record that he or she had been psychiatrically well during follow up with a maximum of one discrete episode lasting less than a year); variable or relapsing remitting (the patient and the case notes report patchy progress with no overall improvement; evidence of relapse and remission with one or more discrete acute episodes lasting more than six months); and chronic (the case notes record almost continuous psychiatric symptoms with one or more episodes lasting over a year).

Descriptive statistics and multiple regression analyses were done with SAS v6.04. Logistic regression analyses were done with EGRET to determine independent factors associated with a course of psychiatric disorder and consultation rate over 11 years.

Results

We traced 87 (90%) subjects at the 11 year follow up. Missing subjects did not differ by sex, diagnosis, or initial severity from those traced but were younger (mean age at follow up 49.5 (95% confidence interval 41.2 to 57.8) years v 60 (56.8 to 63.2) years). Full case note and patient report data were available for 68. Despite the difficulties of recalling past events and the likelihood of present mental state introducing recall bias, there was reasonable agreement between the patients' and general practitioners' records ($\kappa > 0.7$ for serious physical illnesses and major life events such as births and deaths).

Nineteen patients had died. The 11 year standardised mortality ratio for this cohort was 173 (95% confidence interval 164 to 200)

Table 1 Psychiatric and physical course* over 11 years among 68 general practice attenders alive at follow up (values are numbers of patients)

	Psychiatric course	Physical course
Well	22	5
Acute	14	14
Relapsing remitting	20	23
Chronic	12	26

*See text for a definition of outcome groups.

Table 2 Odds ratios for the association between high attendance in primary care and chronic psychiatric course

	Odds ratio (95% confidence interval)	P value
Unadjusted	10.95 (3.13 to 38.3)	< 0.001
Adjusted for age and sex	10.42 (3.03 to 32.89)	< 0.001
Adjusted for age, sex, and chronic physical illness	4.72 (1.12 to 20.28)	< 0.037

compared with 104 for Warwickshire as a whole. The patients who had died were older than survivors (mean age 74.6 (65.9 to 83.2) years v 57.7 (54.5 to 69.8)) but did not differ in sex or initial severity of psychiatric illness. Death was from common causes such as cardiovascular, respiratory, and malignant disease. There were no recorded suicides.

Psychiatric outcome

Of the 68 who returned the 12 item postal general health questionnaire, 35 were classified as cases. Forty seven, however, had lower scores than at one year. Table 1 shows the course of psychiatric and physical illness over the 11 years. Thirty two had a relapsing or chronic psychiatric disorder. Patients with a relapsing course had a mean of 4.9 episodes (median 5, mode 5). Eight of those with a

Continued →

Table 3 Regression coefficients for outcome at 11 years

Outcome variable	Entry variable	Unadjusted R (standard error of estimate)	P value	Adjusted R and (standard error of estimate)	P value
GHQ score	GHQ score	0.42 (0.14)	0.0041	0.38 (0.13)	0.0097
Chronic psychiatric course	GHQ score	0.067 (0.02)	0.0008	0.07 (0.018)	0.0005
Log total consultations	GHQ score	0.28 (0.08)	0.025	0.28 (0.08)	0.019

GHQ – general health questionnaire

chronic course were psychiatrically unwell throughout the follow up period according to case notes and self report. Forty nine had a relapsing or chronic physical illness.

Benzodiazepines were the most commonly prescribed treatment. Sixteen patients received antidepressants at some time, but only one was prescribed an adequate dose.[17] The psychiatric disorders were managed almost exclusively in primary care; there were three referrals to psychiatrists, two to psychologists, and two to social services.

Consultation patterns

The subjects consulted their general practitioners frequently (mean = 115, median = 84, range 0–590 consultations over 11 years). There were no significant differences in consultation rates between the sexes. We defined high attendance as more than 12 visits a year and calculated odds ratios using high attendance as the dependent variable (Table 2). Eighteen patients attended more than 12 times a year over the entire follow up period. Psychiatric illness was independently associated with high attendance after age, sex, and physical illness were adjusted for.

Analysis of general health questionnaire score

Associations between continuous variables at 0, 1, and 11 years were investigated by multiple regression analyses with adjustment for age and sex (Table 3). High initial general health questionnaire score was strongly associated with high general health questionnaire score at 11 years, chronic course of psychiatric illness, and high consultation rates with and without adjustment for age and sex.

We found no association between initial personality assessment or social problems and psychiatric outcomes at 11 years, in contrast to our results at one year. Positive and negative life events recorded by general practitioners in the case notes and reported retrospectively by patients were not associated with psychiatric outcomes, although these are likely to be underreported.

Discussion

Methodological considerations

The cohort was designed to be representative of people attending general practice with common mental disorders. Our results should therefore be generalisable, although it is a small study. Subjects were included only if the general practitioner agreed a psychiatric disorder was present so the results do not apply to patients with hidden morbidity.

The subjects missing at 11 year follow up were younger than the traced subjects.

Continued →

Younger patients may have moved away from the area or their deaths may not have been ascertained.

The 11 year data were obtained from patients retrospectively by postal questionnaire. There was thus a possibility of recall bias and underrecording. However, we also used general practitioners' contemporaneous records over the 11 years to confirm the patients' accounts and classify the course of psychiatric and physical illness. The case notes provide firm data on consultation rate and prescriptions and the analysis has emphasised these.

As general health questionnaire scores were highly correlated with those on the clinical interview schedule ($R = 0.518$, $P < 0.0001$ at recruitment) and as follow up was by post, we thought it was appropriate to send only a general health questionnaire. We recognise, however, the limitations and loss of data incurred by this approach.

Outcomes

The death rate among psychiatric outpatients with neurotic disorders is raised by a factor of 1.5 to 2.0.[14,19] Our findings are consistent with this. Increased deaths have been ascribed to suicide, accidental deaths, or even misdiagnosis of underlying physical conditions, but all our subjects died from common physical disorders.

Our findings support the view that patients with detected neurotic disorders have appreciable illness.[20] Even if the illness was associated with or secondary to physical conditions, we found persistent psychiatric morbidity of a severity that met case criteria after 11 years.

Severity of psychiatric illness at 11 years was associated with severity at entry and one year follow up. A chronic course of psychiatric illness over 11 years was also predicted by initial severity. Social and personality variables were, however, not associated with clinical outcome or course over the 11 years. We had detailed information on social circumstances at entry and one year, case note data during follow up, and retrospective information from the patients after 11 years. None of these data was found to be relevant. However, the sample may have been too small or too homogeneous in addition, little social information was recorded in the general practitioner's notes; a type II error is therefore possible. The problem of statistical power could also account for personality disorder not predicting outcome. Only 31 patients were initially rated as having abnormal personality.

Chronic psychiatric illness was associated with high consultation rates independently of physical illness, age, and sex. All subjects were high users of general practitioner care, and little use was made of other resources.

Conclusions

We did not interfere with the normal management of the patients. After 11 years a large proportion had become chronically unwell high users of primary care services. These findings highlight the need for early identification and prompt and effective treatment of patients with neurotic disorders. The simplest way of identifying this group would be to assess initial severity and morbidity over one year with a simple screening instrument such as the general health questionnaire. Appropriate physical, psychological, and social interventions could then be introduced.[21]

Funding: KL was supported by the Leverhulme Trust.

Conflict of interest: None.

1. Sharp D, Morrell D 1989 The psychiatry of general practice. In: Williams P, Wilkinson G, Rawnsley K, eds. Scientific approaches on epidemiological psychiatry.

Continued →

Essays in honour of Michael Shepherd. London: Routledge, 404–19

2. Shepherd M, Cooper B, Brown A C, Kalson G W, eds. 1966 Psychiatric illness in general practice. London, Oxford University Press

3. Goldberg D, Huxley P 1992 Common mental disorders Routledge: London.

4. Mann A H, Jenkins R, Belsey E 1981 The 12 month outcome of patients with neurotic disorder in general practice. Psychol Med 11: 535–50

5. Tyrer P 1994 Personality disorder. In: Pullen I, Wilkinson G, Wright A, Gray D P, eds. Psychiatry and general practice today: London: Royal Colleges of Psychiatrists and Physicians, 180–93

6. Lloyd K, Jenkins R 1995 The economics of depression in primary care. Br J Psychiatry 66(suppl): 60–2

7. Eisenberg L 1992 Treating depression and anxiety in primary care: closing the gap between knowledge and practice. N Engl J Med 326: 1080–4

8. Corney R, Murray J 1988 The characteristics of high and low attenders at 2 general practices. Social Psychiatry and Psychiatric Epidemiology 23: 39–49

9. Williams P, Wilkinson G, Arreghini E 1989 The determinants of help seeking for psychological disorders in primary health care settings. In: Sartorns N, ed. Psychological disorders in general medical settings. Toronto: Hogrefe and Huber, 21–33

10. Lloyd K 1993 Depression and anxiety among Afro-Caribbean general practice attenders in Britain. Int J Soc Psychiatry 39: 1–9

11. Gerrard T J, Riddell J D 1986 Difficult patients: black holes and secrets. BMJ 98: 530–2

12. Escobar J L, Burnam A 1987 Somatisation in the community. Arch Gen Psychiatry 44: 713–8

13. Goldberg D, Williams P 1988 A user's guide to the general health questionnaire. Windsor: NFER Nelson

14. Goldberg D P, Cooper B, Eastwood M, Kedward H B, Shepherd M 1970 A standardised psychiatric interview for use in community surveys. British Journal of Social and Preventive Medicine 24: 18–23

15. Jenkins R, Mann A H, Belsey E 1981 The background, design and use of a short interview to assess social stress and support in research and clinical settings. Soc Sci Med 15E: 195–203

16. Mann A H, Jenkins R, Cutting J C, Cowen P J 1981 The development and use of a standardised assessment of abnormal personality. Psychiol Med 11: 838–47

17. Paykel E S, Priest R G 1992 Recognition and management of depression in general practice: consensus statement. BMJ 305: 1198–202

18. Sims A 1973 Mortality and neurosis. Lancet ii: 1072–5

19. Sims A, Prior P 1978 The pattern of mortality in severe neuroses. Br J Psychiatry 133: 299–305

20. Dowrick C, Buchan I 1995 Twelve month outcome of depression in general practice: does detection or disclosure make a difference? BMJ 311: 1274–6

21. Lloyd K, Jenkins R 1995 Chronic depression and anxiety in primary care: approaches to liaison. Advances in Psychiatric Treatment 1: 186–90

(Accepted 24 April 1996)

CHAPTER 6

Can the practice introduce an effective strategy to reduce the prescribing of sleeping pills?
An approach to evidence from trials

Irwin Nazareth

Introduction

Many problems presenting to the general practitioner are minor, self-limiting or ill defined; because of this it is sometimes assumed that it is not feasible to use evidence-based medicine in general practice. Yet this view is not substantiated (Ridsdale 1995), and in this chapter I will demonstrate how some of the essential principles of evidence-based medicine can be applied to a clinical situation in the general practice surgery.

The clinical problem

You are a general practice trainee in a three-partner inner London general practice. During the second half of your trainee year, after having had some experience of the running of the surgery, you decide to see if you can implement evidence-based practice. The first patient booked to see you is Ms Smith, a 50-year-old woman who requests a renewal of her 2-monthly repeat prescription for temazepam 20 mg nocte. On reviewing her notes, you discover that she has taken the drug at night, as a sleeping tablet, for the last 10 years. She was first offered the drug as a 'sleeping pill' after an episode of acute back pain which kept her awake for several nights. In the past 10 years, in 1989 and 1992, she has suffered two episodes of depression. Each episode was treated with antidepressants – for 3 months in the first instance and 6 months in the second. There is no other relevant medical history. Having obtained all the necessary information, you make a mental note of the possible management options available for this particular patient. These are:

a. to renew the prescription for the drug without any further intervention
b. to refuse renewal of the prescription and deny the patient further medication
c. to renew the prescription but advise the patient about stopping
d. to consider other possible (published) interventions, currently unknown to you
e. to develop a general practice policy for benzodiazepine prescribing.

Gathering the information

You are not aware of any published information relating to the weaning of patients off benzodiazepines in general practice that could help you to make an evidence-based management decision. You discuss this with your trainer, who suggests you search *Bandolier*: the evidence-based health care journal which is stored in the practice library. *Bandolier* is produced by the *Anglia and Oxford Health Journal* and provides information on recent evidence of clinical interest. On scanning the journal index, you find a reference in the May 1994 issue, which describes a trial of simple strategies used for cutting down on benzodiazepine use by patients in general practice published earlier that year in the *British Journal of General Practice* (Cormack et al 1994). You carry out a manual search of the *British Medical Journal* and the *British Journal of General Practice*, which are stored in the practice library, to identify any other papers published since then. You identify another paper, which describes a trial of brief interventions opportunistically offered by general practitioners to patients using benzodiazepines (Bashir et al 1994). Later that day you decide to do a MEDLINE search using the British Medical Association services via the practice computer. With help from the hospital librarian, you follow the steps outlined by her and conduct a search for publications in the English language under the headings 'benzodiazepines' and 'general practice/family practice'. This does not result in the identification of any other papers.

Description of the interventions proposed

The next step is to read the papers so as to get an overview of the nature of the suggested interventions. The study by Cormack et al (1994) examined the effect of a simple letter requesting the patients to stop using the drug in comparison to a similar letter plus an additional information leaflet from the general practitioner advising patients on how to tackle reduction of benzodiazepine use. A total of 209 long-term users of benzodiazepines were allocated to three groups: 65 to the letter group, 75 to the letter plus information group, and 69 to the control group. After 6 months, both interventions resulted in two-thirds of subjects reducing their intake of medication and 18% receiving no further prescription for the drug, in comparison to the control group.

The paper by Bashir et al (1994) explored the effectiveness of a minimal intervention, offered by the general practitioner to patients using benzodiazepines. General practitioners gave patients opportunistic advice to stop or reduce their use of benzodiazepines. A total of 109 long-term users were recruited, of whom 51 were in the intervention group and the remainder in the control group. Both groups were given a self-help booklet, which was also given to the patients. This strategy resulted in 18% of patients reducing their drug intake.

Both the studies present promising results and hence the next step was to examine the data presented in each of these papers to assess the validity and applicability of this information to clinical practice.

Critical appraisal of the research papers

Both papers can be critically appraised with the help of some of the published guidelines in the 'Users' Guide to Medical Literature' (Guyatt et al 1994a, 1994b). Table 6.1 is a critical review form designed to assess the validity of articles on therapy and is based on the criteria set out in the users' guide. Both papers satisfied most of the criteria (Table 6.1). In the study by Cormack et al, patients were randomly allocated apart from a restriction that they should be similar with respect to age and sex distribution. The method of randomization used in this study, however, was not described. In the study by Bashir et al, allocation to treatment was carried out using odd and even birth dates. Strictly speaking, this method of randomization could be subject to bias and is referred to as systematic allocation. In reality, however, there is no logical explanation as to why groups of subjects born in even years as compared to odd years could be systematically different.

In both studies, blinding of the patient or the general practitioner to the intervention was not possible, as the intervention was an information package or a letter, provided or written by the general practitioner to the patient. The researchers in both the studies may have been blinded, but neither of the papers offered any information on this aspect of design. Lastly, although the composition of the study and control groups at the start of the study was not clearly spelt out in either paper, the information provided in each of the papers suggested that both groups were similar in most respects. One can hence conclude that

Table 6.1 Critical review form for the Cormack et al and Bashir et al studies

Guide	Cormack et al	Bashir et al
I. Are the results valid?		
1. Was the assignment of patients to treatments randomized?	Random but age/sex match method of randomization not indicated	Randomization by odd and even year of birth
2. Were all patients who were entered in the trial properly accounted for and attributed at its conclusion?		
a. Was follow-up complete?	Yes	Yes
b. Were patients analysed in the groups to which they were randomized?	Yes	Yes
3. Were patients, health workers and study personnel 'blind' to treatment?	No	No
4. Were the groups similar at the start of the study?	Information not provided	Information not provided
5. Aside from the experimental intervention, were the groups treated equally?	Yes	Yes
II. What are the results?		
1. How large was the treatment effect?	Table 6.2	Table 6.2
2. How precise was the treatment effect?*	Table 6.2*	Table 6.2*
3. Will the results help me in caring for my patients?	Yes	Yes
a. Can the results be applied to my patient care?	Yes	Yes
b. Were all clinical important outcomes considered?	No	Yes
c. Are the likely benefits worth the potential harms and costs?	Information not provided	Yes

*Refer to the 95% confidence interval as listed in Table 6.2.

within the limitations of the intervention under scrutiny, both trials were adequately designed. Having thus established the validity of the studies, the next step is to use the data provided in both the studies to obtain some idea of the size of effect of each intervention.

How large are the treatment effects?

The treatment effect of an intervention is a measure of the benefit of a treatment. To make an accurate assessment of this, you must compare the outcome data in the intervention group with that of the control group. In this case the two main outcomes of interest are the proportion of subjects who have stopped using the drug 6 months after the interventions and the numbers who have reduced their intake of the drug 6 months after the intervention.

There are several measures that can be calculated from the data provided in the papers. One of these is the likelihood of a patient stopping use of benzodiazepines relative to the controls. This is expressed as the percentage reduction in events treated compared to controls and is known as the relative risk reduction (RRR). Another useful measure is the difference in proportion of patients who stop using benzodiazepines in the intervention and control groups. This is also referred to as the absolute risk reduction (ARR) and is the difference in risk between the treated and control groups.

Lastly, the number of patients who would require an intervention in order to obtain a positive outcome is a very important concept, as it offers clinicians some idea of the effort needed in order to get a good result. It also allows us to make an estimate of the cost of such a service, by calculating how many patients would require an intervention in order to obtain one positive outcome. This is referred to as the numbers needed to treat (NNT) and is calculated as the reciprocal of the absolute risk reduction. It can also be expressed as the numbers of patients requiring treatment during the period of the study in order to prevent one adverse outcome. In both the studies described in this chapter, the numbers needed to treat is the number of patients who would need to receive a letter or receive a minimal intervention from their general practitioner, in order for one of them to stop completely or reduce the use of benzodiazepines within 6 months.

Calculating effects from treatment data

All the measures of treatment effects, as described above, can be easily calculated from the outcome data for each of the interventions described in the papers. The relative risk reduction calculates the proportional reduction in the continued use of benzodiazepines between the intervention and the control group with what would have occurred had there been no treatment. This is done by arithmetic subtraction and division and is expressed as:

C–I/C

where C is the proportion using benzodiazepines in the control group and I is the proportion using benzodiazepines in the intervention group. In the study by Cormack et al, the proportion of patients who had received only a letter and were still using benzodiazepines after 6 months was 0.77 and the proportion on the drug at 6 months who had received both the letter and additional information was 0.87.

In the control group 0.94 continued using the drug. This relative risk reduction is hence calculated:

Letter alone = C–I/C, i.e. 0.94– 0.77/0.94 = 0.181 (expressed as 18.1%)
Letter + information = C–I/C, i.e. 0.94–0.87/0.94 = 0.074 (expressed as 7.4%).

The absolute risk reduction is calculated as the proportional difference in risk between the treated group and the control group. It is expressed as ARR = C–I. Using the proportions from the study by Cormack et al, the calculations for the ARR are:

Letter alone = C–I = 0.94–0.77 = 0.17 (expressed as 17%)
Letter + information = C–I = 0.94–0.87 = 0.07 (expressed as 7%).

Finally, the numbers needed to treat is calculated as the reciprocal of the ARR (i.e. NNT = 1/ARR). Hence in the study by Cormack et al, the NNTs are as follows:

Letter alone = 1/ARR = 1/0.17 = 5.9
Letter + information = 1/ARR = 1/0.07 = 14.3.

Similar calculations have been done using the data provided in the study by Bashir et al (Table 6.2).

The values listed in Table 6.2 provide convincing evidence about the efficacy of the strategies suggested in both trials. Although each of the studies was independently conducted, the relative and absolute risk reduction and the numbers needed to treat in both the trials are very similar. This provides some confirmation of the reliability of the findings. Thus, in the study by Cormack et al, 5.9 patients would need to receive a letter in order to get one patient to stop using benzodiazepines in 6 months. Similarly, in the study by Bashir et al, only 7.7 patients would need to receive an opportunistic intervention from their general practitioner in order for one patient to stop using benzodiazepines. If one were to consider the numbers needed to treat in order for one patient to reduce his or her intake of benzodiazepines, however, only 4.8 patients would need to be sent a letter from their general practitioner (Cormack et al 1994) and only 5.6 would need to receive an opportunistic intervention from a general practitioner in the practice (Bashir et al 1994).

How precise are the treatment effects?

The true value of the risk reduction can never be known: all

Table 6.2 Results form studies: treatment effects

Patient group	Control (C)	Intervention (I)	Relative risk reduction (RRR) with 95% confidence interval RRR = C–I/C	Absolute risk reduction (ARR) with 95% confidence interval ARR = C–I	Numbers of patients needed to treat (NNT) with 95% confidence interval NNT = 1/ARR or = 1/C–I
	I. Routine care study 1 II. Routine care study 2	I. Cormack et al i. Only letter ii. Letter + information pack II. Bashir et al GP intervention			
Patients (%) using benzodiazepines at end of study	I. 94% II. 93%	I i. 77% I ii. 87% II. 80%	I i. 18.1% (3.7–32.4%) I ii. 7.4% (2.7%–17.5%) II. 14% (1–27%)	I i. 17% (2.5–30.5%) I ii. 7% (–2.5–16.5%) II. 13% (1–25%)	I i. 5.9 (3.3–40) I ii. 14.3 (–40–6) II. 7.7 (3.8–50)
Patients using benzodiazepines at same dosage at end of study	I. 84% II. 75%	I i. 63% I ii. 51% II. 57%	I i. 25% (7.7–42.3%) I ii. 39.3% (22.5–56.3%) II. 24% (0.5–47.5%)	I i. 21% (6.5–35.5%) I ii. 33% (18.7–47.3%) II. 18% (0.4–35.6%)	I i. 4.8 (2.8–15.4) I ii. 3 (2.1–5.3) II. 5.6 (2.8–250)

C: Control group (or routine general practice care)
I: Intervention group, 95% confidence intervals

we have is an estimate provided by the two studies and the closest assessment to true treatment effects produced by the trials. Estimates, as derived from the data of the two trials, are unlikely to be precisely correct but the true value would lie somewhere in their neighbourhood. It is possible to identify the range within which this true value may lie 95% of the time by calculating the 95% confidence intervals. This can be done using various statistical software packages. Manual calculations are also possible (Altman 1991). Hence using the data from the study by Cormack et al, 3.3–40 (95% CI, Table 6.2) patients would need to receive a letter in order to get one patient to stop using benzodiazepines in 6 months. Similarly, in the study by Bashir et al, 3.8–50 (95% CI, Table 6.2) patients would need to receive an opportunistic intervention from their general practitioner in order for one patient to stop using benzodiazepines. Thus the true value of the numbers needed to treat in order to stop one patient from using benzodiazepines, would lie somewhere within the range suggested above.

Will the results help me in caring for my patients?

The interventions are valuable, but you need to decide whether the findings are applicable to patients in your practice. Both studies were conducted in British general practices (one was based in London) and most of the patients included in the studies were representative of those seen in daily practice – that is, the exclusion criteria were not excessively rigid. It would therefore seem reasonable to generalize these findings to routine primary care practice in the United Kingdom.

Although the chief outcome of interest is the complete cessation or reduced intake of benzodiazepines, there are other important factors that must be considered prior to implementing a strategy – for example, information on the effects of stopping or reducing medication such as the occurrence of withdrawal symptoms, the effects on the patients' psychological well-being and changes in use of general practice services (i.e. attendance rates) would be required before considering implementation of these findings. A specific search for this information in the two papers reveals that no such data are provided in the study by Cormack et al, whereas this aspect was closely studied in the trial by Bashir et al.

Patients in the intervention group suffered a significantly greater number of withdrawal symptoms than the control group. None of these symptoms, however, resulted in serious complications. Similarly, it was noted that there was no change in the psychiatric status of patients in either the intervention or control groups. Moreover, the service cost as reflected in the general practice consultation rates showed a 11% decrease in those patients receiving opportunistic general practitioner interventions as compared to a 3% decrease in the control group. These values, however, did not reach levels of statistical significance. Finally, it was found that patients on antidepressant therapy at the 6-month follow-up were 10.6 (95% CI 2.0–55.1) times more likely to have reduced their use of benzodiazepines.

Using the evidence to influence your management

The final stage of this process is to use this information in a clinical context. In order to do this, we need to return to the original clinical situation that stimulated this exercise. The evidence from both papers support the two following strategies:

1. Firstly, you could adopt an individual approach in which the patient would be counselled about the dangers of benzodiazepine use by the general practitioner and then offered the self-help leaflet that was used in the study by Bashir et al. This may be combined with a practice policy in which all general practitioners working in the practices would be encouraged to provide a similar opportunistic intervention to all benzodiazepine users. In addition it may be necessary to reassess Ms Smith for symptoms and signs of depression, as this could warrant active antidepressant therapy if one were to use the evidence provided in the study by Bashir et al.

2. Secondly, a wider practice approach to benzodiazepine prescribing could further strengthen the individual approach. This would involve the identification of all patients taking benzodiazepines with the help of practice information systems, followed by the mailing of a letter asking them to cut down their use of the drug. The letter would be designed along the lines of that published in the appendix of the paper by Cormack et al.

It would be important to monitor the outcome of the

intervention by carefully auditing the use of benzodiazepine by the patients in the practice. This would eventually provide data for continuing, modifying or rejecting these strategies for the reduction of benzodiazepine consumption in general practice.

References

Altman D G 1991 Randomisation. British Medical Journal 302: 1481–1482

Bashir K, King M, Ashworth M 1994 Controlled evaluation of brief intervention by general practitioners to reduce chronic use of benzodiazepines. British Journal of General Practice 44: 408–412

Cormack M A, Sweeney K G, Hughes-Jones H, Foot G A 1994 Evaluation of an easy cost-effective strategy for cutting benzodiazepine use in general practice. British Journal of General Practice 44: 5–8

Guyatt G H, Sackett D L, Cook D J 1994a Users' guides to medical literature II. How to use an article about therapy or prevention. A Are the results of the study valid? Journal of the American Medical Association 270: 2598–2601

Guyatt G H, Sackett D L, Cook D J 1994b Users' guides to medical literature II. How to use an article about therapy or prevention. B What were the results and will they help me in caring for my patients? Journal of the American Medical Association 271: 59–63

Ridsdale L 1995 Evidence-based general practice: a critical reader. W B Saunders, London

Sackett D L, Haynes R B, Guyatt G H, Tugwell P 1991 'Deciding on the best therapy' in clinical epidemiology: a basic science for clinical medicine. Little Brown Boston, pp 187–249

© *British Journal of General Practice*, 1994; **44**: 5–8

Evaluation of an easy, cost-effective strategy for cutting benzodiazepine use in general practice

Margaret A Cormack, Kieran G Sweeney, Helen Hughes-Jones, George A Foot

Summary

Aim. This study set out to assess the effect of a letter from the general practitioner, suggesting a reduction in the use of benzodiazepines, and whether the impact of the letter could be increased by the addition of information on how to tackle drug reduction.

Method. Two hundred and nine long-term users of benzodiazepines in general practice were divided into three groups: two intervention groups and a control group. The first intervention group received a letter from their general practitioner asking that benzodiazepine use be gradually reduced and perhaps, in time, stopped. The second intervention group received the same letter plus four information sheets at monthly intervals, designed to assist drug reduction. The mean age of the 209 people was 69 years (age range 34–102 years).

Results. After six months, both intervention groups had reduced their consumption to approximately two thirds of the original intake of benzodiazepines and there was a statistically significant difference between the intervention groups and the control group. Eighteen per cent of those receiving the interventions received no prescriptions at all during the six month monitoring period.

Conclusion. The results indicate that a simple intervention can have a considerable effect on the use of hypnotic and anxiolytic drugs, even with a sample of elderly users.

Keywords

benzodiazepines; drug withdrawal; patient information; patient use of medication; doctor/patient relationship.

Introduction

BENZODIAZEPINE prescribing in the United Kingdom has been falling steadily since the late 1970s, but the number of prescriptions issued is still large: in England in 1989, 21 million prescriptions for hypnotics, sedatives and tranquillizers (as defined by the Department of Health) were issued, the vast majority of these being benzodiazepines.[1] Over time, there has been an increase in the proportion of general practice prescriptions for minor tranquillizers issued on an 'unseen repeat' basis.[2] Characteristically, long-term users of benzodiazepines are older people prescribed hypnotic medication.[3,4]

For over 10 years general practitioners have received clear advice about the problems associated with prescribing benzodiazepines.[5–7] Evidence continues to accumulate that benzodiazepines impair performance, including driving,[8,9] they affect the memory[10] and have adverse cognitive effects.[11] The *British National Formulary* states that hypnotic drugs should be avoided in elderly people, owing to the risks of ataxia and confusion.

M A Cormack, MA. MP PSYCHOL PHD. lecturer in clinical psychology and H Hughes-Jones. BSc. research assistant. Department of Psychology: K G Sweeney, MA MRCGP, research fellow, Department of General Practice: and G A Foot. MA MSc computing development officer. Computing Unit. University of Exeter. Submitted: 22 October 1992; accepted: 8 April 1993

Continued →

A number of studies have assessed the effect of various interventions to reduce the consumption of benzodiazepines. Interventions such as anxiety management, counselling or cognitive therapy have been shown to reduce drug taking.[12–15] Cormack and Sinnott found that a letter from the prescribing general practitioner, advising patients to cut down on their drugs, was as effective as a group run by a psychologist.[16] In a later, controlled study, a similar intervention was found to be as effective as a short consultation with the general practitioner.[17] Both these studies of the effect of a letter from the general practitioner had comparatively small samples of patients, thus limiting the generalizability of the findings. This study, carried out in 1989 and 1990, attempts to assess the effect of such a letter from the prescribing general practitioner to long-term users of benzodiazepines, using a larger sample from the combined populations of three group practices. The effect of the letter is compared with that of a more complex intervention (a series of information sheets) and with the results from a control group who received no intervention.

Method

Design
Long-term regular users of benzodiazepines were defined as patients who were receiving at least one prescription for benzodiazepines every two months and had taken benzodiazepines continuously for at least six months. Long-term users were identified by general practitioners and divided into three groups: two intervention groups and a control group. Within each doctor's list, identified users were allocated to the three groups, roughly matched for age and sex to ensure a representative spread between groups. Beyond this, allocation to groups was random and was performed by the research assistant (H H-J).

Those in intervention group one received a letter from their general practitioner asking them to try to reduce or stop their benzodiazepine medication and advising that this should be done gradually (Appendix 1). Intervention group two received the same letter, followed at monthly intervals by four information sheets giving advice about reducing medication, including practical suggestions for coping without drugs. The control group received no intervention. Prescriptions issued to all groups were monitored for six months. After six months, the control group was offered the more successful intervention.

Sample
The sample was drawn from three group practices with three or four general practitioners and approximately average list size in a city in the south west of England. All the doctors in the practices were already trying to prevent the long-term use of benzodiazepines through discussion of the drugs with their patients. Ten general practitioners with personal lists in the three practices were asked to identify long-term regular users of benzodiazepines. Individuals were identified from their repeat prescribing records, either manually recorded or computer generated. The criteria for exclusion were that the patient was in a current crisis or with an illness for which the drugs were required at the time, had a current diagnosis of psychosis or dementia, was in a position where a hospital doctor or a carer could administer medication, was known to abuse alcohol or was unable to read.

Analysis
In order to compare individuals benzodiazepine consumption, a calculation of equivalent doses for the various drugs

Continued →

prescribed was made. Diazepam 5 mg was considered as one tablet and equivalents were calculated according to the recommended dosages cited in the *British National Formulary*, with advice from a pharmacist.

A baseline benzodiazepine use was established for each patient by taking all the prescriptions issued in the year prior to the date of sending the letter and dividing the total number of tablet equivalents by two (one year of baseline could be considered as all participants in the study had been taking benzodiazepines for at least a year). By considering one whole year, any seasonal variations in prescribing were avoided. Benzodiazepine use in the six months prior to the intervention was also measured as a second baseline to allow for the possibility that the patients were already reducing the drugs they were taking immediately prior to the intervention (without this, reduction could have been misattributed to the intervention).

Because the data from the records were in terms of prescriptions issued, which is only an approximate measure of consumption, a more accurate calculation of tablet consumption was devised. Prescriptions issued just before the time of the intervention would have been consumed partly in the baseline periods and partly in the monitoring period. Prescriptions issued before the beginning of the baseline periods and before the end of the monitoring period would have been only partly consumed during these periods. It was assumed that during the baseline periods the drugs were taken at a regular rate. The amount of the prescription issued prior to the intervention date which would have been consumed at the baseline rate was calculated and the rest of the prescription was allocated to the monitoring period (in cases where people did not have further prescriptions, that is, they responded to the request to stop, this procedure may have overestimated the consumption in the

monitoring period). A similar process was undertaken to calculate the amount of a prescription consumed at the end of the monitoring period. Again, this may have led to an overestimate of the drugs consumed as there could have been a gradual reduction throughout the monitoring period. Given that any errors of overestimation would have detracted from finding a significant result attributable to the intervention, the procedure was felt to be satisfactory.

One-way analysis of variance and tests were used to compare tablet consumption between the groups.

Results

A total of 268 people were identified as long-term regular users of benzodiazepines. Fifty nine were excluded from analysis by H H-J – five were incorrectly identified, six had incomplete records, seven died before or during the study, six left the practice before or during the study, 23 fulfilled the exclusion criteria before or during the study and 12 stopped taking benzodiazepines before the study. There was no evidence to suggest a link between the intervention and death or leaving the practice. Thus, 209 people provided data for analysis. The characteristics of the sample are shown in Table 1.

Participants in the study were allocated to the three groups and the result was: letter group, 65 people: letter plus information group, 75; and control group, 69. The discrepancy in numbers between the groups arose by chance, mostly owing to exclusion from the trial after the start.

The number of tablet equivalents taken in the monitoring period was divided by the number taken during the baseline period for each patient in the study (Table 2). The intervention groups reduced to

Continued →

Table 1 Characteristics of the sample of 209 people.

Median age (years)	71
Mean age (years)	69
Age range (years)	34–102
Number of women	166
Number of men	43
Ratio of women:men	4:1
Number of people taking:	
One benzodiazepine	177
Two or more benzodiazepines	32
Anxiolytics only	67
Hypnotics only	119
Anxiolytics and hypnotics	23
Median (range):	
Duration of any benzodiazepine use (years)	15 (1–29)
Duration of continuous benzodiazepine use (years)	9 (1–29)
Number of non-benzodiazepine drugs currently taken	6 (0–31)

Table 2 Effect of the interventions on benzodiazepine consumption.

Group	Mean[a] (95% confidence interval)	
Monitoring period divided by baseline consumption		
Letter (n = 65)	0.68	(0.57 to 0.78)
Letter + information (n = 75)	0.63	(0.53 to 0.72)
Control (n = 69)	0.90	(0.80 to 1.01)
	$F = 8.54$: 2, 206 df; $P<0.001$	
Monitoring period divided by consumption in the six months prior to intervention		
Letter (n = 65)	0.71	(0.59 to 0.83)
Letter + information (n = 75)	0.64	(0.54 to 0.75)
Control (n = 69)	0.93	(0.83 to 1.03)
	$F = 7.63$; 2, 206 df; $P<0.001$	

n = number of people in group, df = degrees of freedom.
[a]Mean of number of tablet equivalents taken in the monitoring period divided by the number taken during the baseline period / six month period prior to intervention for each person.

Table 3 Patterns of reduction of benzodiazepine use.

	% of people	
Group	With no prescriptions after intevention date	Who reduced to half or less of original consumption
Letter (n = 65)	23	37
Letter + information (n = 75)	13	49
Control (n = 69)	6	16

n = number of people in group.

approximately two thirds of their original intake and there was a statistically significant difference in the reductions of the three groups. A t-test was performed to determine whether one intervention was more effective than the other and no significant difference was found between the interventions.

Comparison of consumption in the monitoring period and in the six months immediately preceding the intervention produced similar results, but with slightly higher proportions (Table 2). Again, the three groups were significantly different and there was no difference between the intervention groups.

Table 3 shows the pattern of reduction of benzodiazepine use in the three groups. For a proportion of people, the long-term use of benzodiazepines can be stopped completely by a simple intervention from the general practitioner.

There were no sex differences in the degree of success, nor were there differences between the practices. The numbers were too small for comparison of individual general practitioners to be made.

Age correlated negatively with the proportion of tablets taken after the intervention date compared with the baseline period ($r = -0.26$. $P < 0.01$). This indicated that older people did a little better in reducing their consumption than younger people.

Continued →

Although this is a significant result, the correlation coefficient is fairly small, and there would be little clinical significance attached to this finding.

The number of different benzodiazepines taken did not affect the degree of success at reducing drug consumption. Similarly, success was not related to whether the drugs were taken as anxiolytics or hypnotics.

Discussion

Twelve people from the original 268 (4.5%) had stopped taking benzodiazepines in the few months between identification as suitable research participants and the start of the study, and there was also an overall reduction of 10% in drug use for the people in the control group. These figures indicate that a small proportion of people do discontinue or reduce benzodiazepine use after taking the tablets regularly for some time. One reason for reduction may be the influence of the media, but the figures may also reflect the routine work of the doctors in the study in discussing tablet use during consultations.

The study demonstrated that older people are just as good, if not better, than younger people at reducing their consumption of benzodiazepines and thus it is well worth trying to help these people to stop taking their drugs. It is not known whether longterm use of benzodiazepines constituted dependence for the patients in the sample, but the finding that older people did better than younger ones matches the finding of Schweizer and colleagues that elderly people (over 60 years of age) suffered from a less severe withdrawal syndrome from benzodiazepines than their younger counterparts.[18] The adverse effects of the drugs are greater in older populations and smaller doses are necessary.[19] There is thus every reason to encourage older users to reduce medication in order to prevent the unwanted effects of the drugs.

In the sample studied here, the ratio of women to men was 4:1. This ratio is higher than in most other studies, which report a ratio of approximately 2:1.[4,20] This could be explained by the predominately elderly status of the population, which would be primarily female. Within the group of older women, there are two obvious sub-groups: one may have been prescribed benzodiazepines for bereavement, the other may be a cohort of women who commenced benzodiazepine use at the menopause many years before, as the drugs were used extensively to treat menopausal symptoms.[21]

Nearly twice as many people were taking benzodiazepines as hypnotic drugs as were taking them as anxiolytic drugs. The research literature and media coverage of the use of benzodiazepines have focused on anxiolytics rather than hypnotics. This study has shown that when intervention is aimed at reducing anxiolytic and hypnotic drugs, success can be achieved with both.

It was interesting to note that there was no evidence of a difference in the effectiveness of the interventions. The information sheets had been produced because previous research[17] had shown that people did not have well-formed strategies when they set about reducing medication. The content of the information sheets had been pre-tested and found to be easy to read and assimilate. Despite this, the information failed to enhance the effect of the initial letter. There was no feedback to the doctors to suggest any reasons for the lack of effectiveness of the information sheets.

This study has two important findings. First, it consolidates the position of a minimum intervention – a doctor's letter – as an effective tool in reducing the consumption of benzodiazepines. Secondly, it demonstrates that a more complex, costly,

Continued →

and time consuming intervention is no more effective.

The implications of these findings are twofold. First, associated with the reduction in consumption is a reduction in iatrogenic morbidity. This is particularly important in elderly people, the largest group using these drugs in this study, in whom confusion and ataxia are associated with these drugs (*British national formulary*). Large numbers of people who have taken these drugs over long periods of time complain of the ill effects of the drugs, and legal action is now being taken against drug companies and doctors who prescribed the drugs. Dependence on benzodiazepines is an important problem and there are indications of cognitive impairments, possibly linked to brain damage, through the protracted use of benzodiazepines.[22] The quality of life of many people could be greatly improved by stopping continuous, regular use of these drugs.

Secondly, in England in 1989, nearly nine million prescriptions for sedatives and tranquillizers and over 12 million prescriptions for hypnotics were issued from family health services.[1] The total cost of these prescriptions was nearly £34 million. Assuming, as a conservative estimate, that at least 80% of the prescriptions were for benzodiazepine preparations, the total cost of benzodiazepine prescriptions would have been over £27 million. If, as has been suggested,[20] half of the prescriptions issued in any year go to long-term users, and if a 30% reduction in drug use can be expected by sending a letter to long-term users, then a drugs saving of at least £4 million at 1989 prices could be achieved.

The drug reduction of 30% found here was achieved with a hard core of patients who had had repeated advice from their general practitioners to reduce their medication and who had not responded to these more informal overtures. With other patient populations, who may have had little

expression of concern about drug use from their general practitioners, it may be expected that an even greater response would occur.

Why is the letter from the doctor effective? It may have been that the letter reached a sub-group of the benzodiazepine consumers who were ambivalent about taking the drugs, and needed a final stimulus to stop, rather like the sub-group of smokers, who need a similar sharp stimulus to increase their will-power.[23] The power of the letter is another illustration of the therapeutic potential of the doctor-patient relationship, first described by Michael Balint in his classic text.[24]

Are there any other clinical situations in which this kind of intervention might be used? The use of prochlorperazine in small doses in elderly people has been shown to be at best marginally effective, and at worst a source of serious side effects, namely extrapyramidal symptoms.[25] This could be a possible target for this kind of intervention.

As far as the consumption of benzodiazepines is concerned, the situation is now quite clear. If all general practitioners in the UK wrote to their long-term benzodiazepine users about trying to reduce drug consumption, then there would be a substantial reduction in the morbidity associated with their side effects, as well as a considerable saving in the drugs bill.

Appendix 1. Letter from general practitioner received by intervention groups.

Dear …

I am writing to you because I note from our records that your have been taking … for some time now. Recently, family doctors have become concerned about this kind of tranquillizing medication when it is taken over long periods. Our concern is that the body can get used to these tablets so that they no longer work properly. If you stop taking the tablets suddenly, there may be unpleasant

Continued →

withdrawal effects which you will experience. Research work done in this field shows that repeated use of the tablets over a long time is no longer recommended. More importantly, these tablets may actually cause anxiety and sleeplessness and they can be addictive.

I am writing to ask you to consider cutting down on your dose of these tablets and perhaps stopping them at some time in the future. The best way to do this is to take the tablets only when you feel they are absolutely necessary. Try to take them only when you know that you have to do something that might be difficult for you. In this way you might be able to make a prescription last longer.

Once you have begun to cut down, you might be able to think about stopping them altogether. It would be best to cut down very gradually and then you will be less likely to have withdrawal symptoms.

If you would like to talk to me personally about this, I would be delighted to see you in the surgery whenever it is convenient for you to attend.

Yours sincerely

References

1. Department of Health. 1991 Health and personal social services statistics for England. London: HMSO
2. Williams P, Bellantuono C 1991 Long-term tranquilliser use: the contribution of epidemiology. In: Gabe J (ed). Understanding tranquilliser use. London: Routledge
3. Rodrigo E K, King M B, Williams P 1988 Health of long-term benzodiazepine users. BMJ 296: 603–606
4. Dunbar G C, Perera M H, Jenner F A 1989 Patterns of benzodiazepine use in Great Britain as measured by a general population survey. Br J Psychiatry 155: 836–841
5. Committee on the Review of Medicines 1980 Systematic review of the benzodiazepines. BMJ 280: 910–912
6. Committee on Safety of Medicines 1988 Benzodiazepines, dependence and withdrawal symptoms. Current Problems 21
7. The Royal College of Psychiatrists 1988 Benzodiazepines

and dependence: a College statement. Bull R Coll Psychiatrists 12: 107–108
8. Hindmarch I 1981 Psychotropic drugs and psychomotor performance. In: Murray R, Ghodse H, Harris C, et al (eds). The misuse of psychotropic drugs. London: Gaskell The Royal College of Psychiatrists
9. Prescott L F 1983 Safety of the benzodiazepines. In: Costa E (ed). The benzodiazepines from molecular biology to clinical practice. New York, NY: Raven Press
10. Bixler E O, Kales A, Manfredi R L 1991 et al. Next-day memory impairment with triazolam use. Lancet 337: 827–831
11. Golombok S, Moodley P, Lader M H 1988 Cognitive impairment in long-term benzodiazepine users. Psychol Med 18: 365–374
12. Giblin M J, Clift A D 1983 Sleep without drugs. J R Coll Gen Pract 33: 628–633
13. Skinner P T 1984 Skills not pills: learning to cope with anxiety symptoms. J R Coll Gen Pract 34: 258–260
14. Higgitt A, Golombok S, Fonagy P, Lader M 1987 Group treatment of benzodiazepine dependence. Br J Addiction 82: 517–532
15. Jones D 1991 Weaning elderly patients off psychotropic drugs in general practice: a randomised controlled trial. Health Trends 22: 164–166
16. Cormack M A, Sinnott A 1983 Psychological alternatives to long-term benzodiazepine use. J R Coll Gen Pract 33: 279–281
17. Cormack M A, Owens R G, Dewey M E 1989 The effect of minimal interventions by general practitioners on long-term benzodiazepine use. J R Coll Gen Pract 39: 408–411
18. Schweizer E, Case G, Rickels K 1989 Benzodiazepine dependence and withdrawal in elderly patients. Am J Psychiatry 146: 529–531
19. Morgan K 1983 Sedative-hypnotic drug use and ageing. Arch Geronto Geriatr 2: 181–199
20. Ashton H, Golding J F 1989 Tranquillisers prevalence, predictors and possible consequences. Data from a large United Kingdom survey. Br J Addition 84: 541–546
21. Parry H J, Balter M B, Mellinger G D 1973 et al. National patterns of psychotherapeutic drug use. Arch Gen Psychiatry 28: 769–783
22. Lader M H, Ron M, Petursson H 1984 Computed axial brain tomography in long-term benzodiazepine users. Psychol Med 14: 203–206
23. Russell M A H, Wilson C, Taylor C, Baker C D 1979 Effect of general practitioners' advice against smoking. BMJ 2: 231
24. Balint M 1964 The doctor, his patient and the illness. London: Pitman
25. Ramsden R T 1992 Balance disorders in the elderly. Med Dialogue 351: 1–2

Continued →

Acknowledgements

The study was funded by a grant from the Devon Northcott Medical Foundation and by a contribution from the Department of Clinical and Community Psychology, Exeter Health Authority. Rachel Kirby gave computer expertise, Sandy Salisbury provided secretarial services, Karen Jackson typed the various stages of the manuscript, Stuart Brooks helped in the initial programming of the database and Ann-Marie Corner assisted in the data entry onto the computer. The University of Exeter Departments of Psychology and General Practice collaborated on this joint venture and encouraged the development of the research. The doctors in the study took part in the planning and design stages and we would like to thank them and their practice staff for their continuing help in the data collection.

Address for correspondence

Dr M A Cormack, Wessex Regional Training Course in Clinical Psychology, Knowle Hospital, Fareham, Hampshire PO17 5NA.

© *British Journal of General Practice* 1994: **44**, 408–412.

Controlled evaluation of brief intervention by general practitioners to reduce chronic use of benzodiazepines

Khaver Bashir, Michael King, Mark Ashworth

SUMMARY

Background. It is recommended that long-term users of benzodiazepines in general practice be withdrawn from their medication where possible.

Aim. A study was undertaken to assess the effectiveness of minimal intervention delivered by general practitioners in helping chronic users of benzodiazepines to withdraw from their medication, and to determine the psychological sequelae on patients of such intervention.

Method. Patients taking benzodiazepines regularly for at least one year were recruited by their general practitioner and allocated either to a group receiving *brief advice* during one consultation supplemented by a *self-help booklet* or to a control group who received routine care. The patients completed the 12-item general health questionnaire and a benzodiazepine withdrawal symptom questionnaire at the outset of the study and at three and six months after this.

Results. Eighteen per cent of patients in the intervention group (9/50) had a reduction in benzodiazepine prescribing recorded in the notes compared with 5% of the 55 patients in the control group ($P < 0.05$). In the intervention group, 63% of patients had a score of two or more on the general health questionnaire at baseline compared with 52% at six months. Of the 20 intervention patients reporting benzodiazepine reduction, 60% had a score of two or more at baseline compared with 40% at six months. Intervention patients had significantly more qualitative, but not quantitative, withdrawal symptoms at six months compared with baseline. Consultation rates were not increased in the intervention group.

Conclusion. The study indicates that some chronic users can successfully reduce their intake of benzodiazepines with simple advice from the general practitioner and a self-help booklet. This type of intervention does not lead to psychological distress or increased consultation.

Keywords
benzodiazepines; drug long-term use; drug dependence; drug addiction treatment.

Introduction

Benzodiazepine prescribing in the United Kingdom reached a peak in 1979 with 31 million prescriptions being dispensed.[1] Since then there has been a decline, mainly as a result of a drop in new prescribing,[2] leaving a core of chronic users who are treated in general practice. In 1988, the Committee on Safety of Medicines recommended that benzodiazepines should not be used for more than four weeks and then only at the lowest possible dose to control symptoms.[3] Previous studies have indicated that many chronic users are elderly, and even as early as 1980 the Committee on the Review of Medicines had noted the increased frequency of adverse

K Bashir, MRCGP, research fellow and M King, MD, PhD, MRCP, FRCGP, MRCPsych, senior lecturer, Academic Department of Psychiatry, Royal Free Hospital School of Medicine, London. M Ashworth, MRCGP, general practitioner, London.

Submitted: 20 April 1993; accepted: 2 November 1993.

Continued →

reactions in this group, particularly among those taking long acting preparations.[4] A report published in 1992 includes a recommendation that primary care teams should identify long-term users of benzodiazepines on their list and, where possible, plan their withdrawal from medication.[5] However, in the context of general practice where consultations often last no more than 10 minutes, only brief intervention is really feasible. Previous work has shown that a proportion of long-term users can successfully decrease or stop taking their benzodiazepines in response to a letter from or a short interview with their general practitioner.[6,7]

A study was undertaken to investigate whether general practitioner minimal intervention, consisting of brief advice plus a self-help booklet, could help chronic users to withdraw from their benzodiazepines. A further aim was to measure the levels of psychological distress experienced before and after intervention to see if there was any change.

Method

Eleven volunteer general practices in the London area took part in the study. General practitioners were asked to recruit all chronic benzodiazepine users by writing to patients receiving repeat prescriptions and asking them to attend the surgery. When they attended the project was explained and informed consent obtained. Doctors also recruited patients opportunistically if they happened to attend during the trial period.

A chronic user was defined as someone who had been on benzodiazepines for at least a year and who took tablets at least three times weekly. The following patients were excluded: those with acute serious illness; anyone currently receiving psychiatric treatment or with a history of psychosis; anyone currently dependent on alcohol or

illicit drugs; patients taking benzodiazepines for a medical problem such as epilepsy; patients unable to attend the surgery because of physical infirmity; and individuals unable to complete questionnaires for any reason. General practitioners were also allowed to exclude a chronic user if they felt that asking such a patient to reduce their benzodiazepines might be harmful (the doctor kept a list of this group).

Patients were allocated by their doctor to receive either minimal intervention, consisting of general practitioner advice on coming off benzodiazepines plus a self-help booklet which patients took away to read, or to receive no intervention: this group acted as controls. The birth date method was used to allocate patients (individuals having an even birth date received minimal intervention while those with an odd birth date received no intervention).

It would have been impossible in a controlled trial to impose rigid guidelines on general practitioners concerning the management of benzodiazepine withdrawal. Instead it was suggested that doctors should outline the risks of benzodiazepines, advise patients to reduce and then stop their medication, and then encourage patients to follow the advice in the self-help booklet. The booklet was divided into two sections, the first giving some basic information about benzodiazepines and the second giving practical advice on stopping, including techniques on coping with fears and anxieties. It had been specifically designed for the study and had already been successfully used in a pilot study with 31 patients.[8]

Assessment

The main research instruments were the 12-item general health questionnaire[9] which is used to screen for psychiatric disorder in

Continued →

general practice populations, and the benzodiazepine withdrawal questionnaire[10] which measures quantitative perceptual symptoms (hyper- or hypo-sensitivity in sensory modalities) and qualitative perceptual phenomena (such as strange or unusual tastes or smells), giving an estimate of the level of withdrawal symptoms being experienced by the patient.

Subjects completed these questionnaires at the initial consultation and were posted the same questionnaires three and six months later. General practitioners kept a list of patients who were unwilling to complete the baseline questionnaires; these patients were considered to be study refusals and so were not entered into the controlled trial. At six months subjects reported whether their consumption of benzodiazepines had increased, stayed the same, decreased or stopped during the previous six months. Factors considered by patients to have either assisted or prevented reduction were also noted.

All patients' records (study patients, refusals and those chronic users specifically excluded from the study by their doctor) were examined at six months to ascertain benzodiazepine prescribing, consultation rates, past medical and psychiatric histories and details of other drugs prescribed. Benzodiazepine dosages were expressed in terms of diazepam equivalents using the conversion table in the 1989 *British National Formulary*, number 18. With some computers if the doctor wishes to prescribe more tablets than usual a multiple prescription is issued (for example, three prescriptions of 30 tablets of temazepam 10 mg rather than one prescription of 90 tablets). However, the same multiple entry can appear owing to computer error (for example, failure to print a prescription until the third attempt). This type of problem was encountered in four of the 11 practices. All multiple entries, which could not be checked against manual records,

were taken at face value. This may have led to an overestimate in a few cases, though such errors should have been equally distributed between control and intervention patients. In view of this problem strict criteria were used to define reduction, namely the mean daily dose being reduced by a minimum of 5 mg diazepam equivalent or by at least 75% in the six months following intervention compared with the six months prior to intervention. Henceforth reduction defined in this way will be referred to as recorded reduction; reported reduction will refer to patients who reported decreasing or stopping their benzodiazepines at six months; reported stopping will refer to patients who reported stopping their benzodiazepines at six months (those reporting stopping are thus a subgroup of those reporting a reduction).

Doctors were interviewed at the end of the trial to determine their attitudes to benzodiazepines, particularly in relation to short- and long-term prescribing, and litigation issues. The interviews were conducted by K B and consisted of a series of closed questions.

Analysis

Based on previous research[6] it was assumed that if 30% of the intervention subjects and 5% of the controls reduced their drug consumption, this would constitute a clinically significant difference. In order to demonstrate this difference with 90% power and at the 0.05 level of significance, it was estimated that 47 subjects were required in each group.[11]

Intervention and control patients were compared for levels of recorded reduction, reported reduction and reported stopping. There is now considerable evidence supporting a separate classification of chronic daytime and night-time users of benzodiazepines.[12] Therefore levels of

Continued →

reduction among intervention and control patients were also calculated for day- and night-time users (patients taking benzodiazepines both during the day and at night were considered daytime users).

General health questionnaire and withdrawal questionnaire scores were compared between baseline and six months, and consultation rates compared for the six months before and after baseline in the control group, intervention group and two subgroups of the intervention group – those reporting reduction and those reporting no reduction. By looking at the data from the whole intervention group it was possible to answer the question 'Does asking chronic users to withdraw from benzodiazepines lead to psychological distress, withdrawal symptoms or increased consultation?' The data relating to intervention patients reporting reduction or non-reduction allowed two further questions to be answered 'Does asking chronic users to withdraw from benzodiazepines lead to psychological distress, withdrawal symptoms or increased consultation when the patient reports reduction and when the patient reports no reduction?'

Comparisons were assessed using chi square tests and *t*-tests. Non-parametric tests were used for non-normal variables. Logistic regression was performed to determine independent predictors of recorded reduction of benzodiazepines, reported reduction and reported stopping (the forward stepwise method was used; continuous independent variables were dichotomized around their medians). Independent variables were chosen from previous research or clinical experience which indicated that they might be important: some related to benzodiazepines (baseline dosage, during of action, years on medication and day- or night-time use); others to patients (sex, marital status and social class); and others to doctors (age and levels of short- and long-term

benzodiazepine prescribing) or their practices (single-handed or group practices, and attachment of mental health professionals).

Results

Characteristics of study population

One hundred and nine chronic users were recruited into the study, most during the first half of 1991. Fifty one (47%) were in the intervention group. The mean age of the sample was 62 years (range 32 to 86 years). Sixty seven (61%) were women. Twenty three participants were single, 32 were married, and 47 were divorced, separated or widowed (marital status of seven patients unknown).

The mean duration of treatment with benzodiazepines was 14 years (range two to 26 years). At the start of the study 30 patients were taking diazepam, 24 nitrazepam, 44 temazepam, 13 lorazepam, three oxazepam and one triazolam (some patients were taking more than one benzodiazepine; data missing for one patient). Seventy three subjects took their benzodiazepine at night-time only, 16 during the day only and 20 both at night and during the day. According to the patient records the general practitioner had been the first to prescribe a benzodiazepine in 89 (82%) cases, a psychiatrist in seven and another doctor in a further seven (in six cases the original prescriber was unknown). The initial prescription was for an overtly psychological reason in 57 patients, for a physical problem (most often headache or some other regional pain) in 19 patients and for reasons unknown in the remaining 33 cases. Based only on data in the notes the median number of attempts to withdraw from benzodiazepines prior to the present study was one (range zero to seven).

Fifty four patients (50%) had seen a psychiatrist at some point. Forty seven (43%)

Continued →

had been treated for depression and 21 (19%) for anxiety by someone other than the general practitioner. Thirty patients had a history of alcohol problems and 18 had attempted suicide at least once. In terms of their physical health, 44 had suffered a major cardiovascular or vascular episode, 40 a major respiratory illness and 40 a major gastrointestinal illness. The median number of major physical diseases per patient was three.

Refusals and exclusions by general practitioners

Sixteen patients had been considered to be refusals as they had not been willing to complete the baseline questionnaires and a further 14 had been excluded by their general practitioner. Those refusing to take part did not differ significantly from the study sample in terms of age, sex, physical or psychiatric health, consultation rate in the six months before the study or benzodiazepine prescribing history. Those excluded by the general practitioner were more likely than the study patients to be on an antidepressant at the end of the trial period; seven of those excluded (50%) were on an antidepressant compared with 18 (17%) of the study patients (Fisher exact test, 1 degree of freedom (df), 2 tailed $P<0.01$; 95% confidence interval (CI) for difference between proportions 6% to 61%).

Response to questionnaires

The general health questionnaire and withdrawal questionnaire were completed by all 109 patients at baseline, by 89% at three months, and by 85% at six months. The 16 non-respondents at six months comprised two who had died, one who had spent much time in hospital, eight who declined to fill in the second or third questionnaires and five who were not contactable. Ninety of the 93 respondents at six months also reported on their consumption of benzodiazepines over the previous six months.

Table 1 Prevalence of psychiatric disorder in study sample at baseline, three and six months according to different case thresholds on the general health questionnaire.

	% of patients who are		
	Mild cases[a]	Moderate cases[b]	Severe cases[c]
Baseline ($n = 109$)	55	47	35
3 months ($n = 97$)	49	42	38
6 months ($n = 93$)	46	37	33

n = number of patients in group. [a]Score of 2+. [b]Score of 3+. [c]Score of 4+.

Table 1 shows the prevalence of psychiatric disorder in the study population using three different case thresholds on the general health questionnaire. At baseline 55% of subjects were mild cases (a score of two or more) and 35% severe cases (four or more), while at six months 46% were mild cases and 33% severe cases. The 16 non-respondents to the final general health questionnaire did not differ significantly in terms of caseness from the rest of the study sample at baseline.

Recorded and reported benzodiazepine reduction

Benzodiazepine prescribing data were collected for 105 patients (two patients died during follow up and for two cases full prescribing records were not available for the six months before and after intervention). Of these 105 patients 50 (48%) were in the intervention group. Nine (18%) of the intervention group had a recorded reduction in benzodiazepine prescription compared with three (5%) of the control group ($\chi^2 = 4.07$, 1 df, $P<0.05$: 95% CI for difference between proportions 0.3% to 25%). Among the 71 night-time users, a recorded reduction

Continued →

was achieved by eight of 33 in the intervention group (24%) compared with two (5%) of the 38 in the control group (Fisher exact test, 1 df, two tailed $P<0.05$; 95% CI for difference between proportions 3% to 35%). Among the 34 day-time users, a recorded reduction was achieved by one patient out of 17 (6%) in each of the control and intervention groups.

Of the 90 patients who reported their benzodiazepine consumption at the end of the six month follow up 46 (51%) were in the intervention group. Twenty of the intervention group (43%) reported a reduction in intake of benzodiazepines compared with 11 (25%) of the controls (difference not significant). Nine of the intervention group (20%) reported stopping taking their benzodiazepines compared with three of the controls (7%) (difference not significant). Among the 62 night-time users, a reported reduction was achieved by 17 of the 32 in the intervention group (53%) compared with seven (23%) of the 30 in the control group ($\chi^2 = 5.79$, 1 df, $P<0.05$; 95% CI for difference between proportions 7% to 53%). Among the 28 day-time users, a reported reduction was achieved by three of 14 in the intervention group (21%) compared with four (29%) of 14 in the control group (difference not significant).

Although not measuring precisely the same thing, the level of agreement between recorded and self-report data was examined: for a comparison of recorded and reported reduction kappa = 0.34; for recorded reduction and reported stopping kappa = 0.61. The strict criteria used to define recorded reduction made it much closer to reported stopping than to a measure of reported reduction.

Questionnaire scores and consultation rates
Intervention and control patients. The proportion of patients who were cases according to the general health questionnaire was lower at six months compared with baseline in both intervention and control group patients (Table 2). The fall was more pronounced in the intervention group (11%) than in the control group (3%), though neither reached significance. Intervention patients had significantly more qualitative (but not quantitative) withdrawal symptoms at six months compared with baseline. In the control group both qualitative and quantitative symptoms were unchanged over the six months. A comparison of the median number of consultations in the six months before and after intervention revealed no significant difference in the control group (four and four, respectively) or the intervention group (four and three, respectively).

Intervention patients reporting benzodiazepine reduction and non-reduction. Intervention patients reporting a reduction in benzodiazepine consumption and those reporting no reduction both had a lower proportion of patients who were cases according to the general health questionnaire at six months compared with baseline (Table 2). The fall was greater among the reducers (20%) than in the non-reducers (3%), though neither reached significance. Both subgroups had significantly more qualititative (but not quantitative) withdrawal symptoms at six months compared with baseline. A comparison of the median number of consultations in the six months before and after intervention revealed no significant difference among either reducers (2.5 and 3.5, respectively) or non-reducers (four and three, respectively).

The nine intervention patients reporting a reduction who actually stopped taking benzodiazepines showed no improvement in psychiatric status (six were cases according to

Continued →

Table 2 Prevalence of psychiatric morbidity, according to general health questionnaire, and withdrawal symptoms among intervention and control group patients, and among intervention patients reporting reduction and no reduction in benzodiazepine consumption, at baseline and at six months.

| | No. (%) of GHQ cases[a] | | Withdrawal symptom score | | | |
| | | | Qualitative (mean (SD)) | | Quantitative (median) | |
	Baseline	6 months	Baseline	6 months	Baseline	6 months
Intervention group	29 (63)	24 (52)	5.5 (5.8)	7.3 (6.2)**	1	0
Control group	20 (43)	19 (40)	4.8 (4.5)	5.7 (5.9)	1	0.5
Intervention group						
Reducers	12 (60)	8 (40)	6.4 (6.9)	8.6 (6.6)*	0	1.5
Non-reducers	17 (65)	16 (62)	4.9 (4.8)	6.2 (5.8)*	1	0

[a]Score of 2+. Paired *t*-test: *$P<0.05$, **$P<0.01$.

the general health questionnaire at baseline and six were cases at six months). Among the intervention 11 patients reporting decreasing but not stopping benzodiazepines, six were cases at baseline compared with two at six months.

Logistic regression

Two factors were found to be associated with recorded reduction of benzodiazepines: being on an antidepressant at the end of the six month follow up (odds ratio 10.6, 95% CI 2.0 to 55.1) and being a member of the intervention group (odds ratio 6.0, 95% CI 1.1 to 32.5).

Two factors emerged as being predictive of reported reduction in the study population: taking a low baseline dose of benzodiazepine, that is, 4.5 mg daily or less of diazepam equivalent (odds ratio 3.8, 95% CI 1.3 to 10.8) and being on a short acting drug, such as temazepam, oxazepam, lorazepam or triazolam (odds ratio 4.1, 95% CI 1.4 to 11.9). Having a history of four or more major physical illnesses was an independent predictor of reported stopping (odds ratio 4.7, 95% CI 1.1 to 19.5).

No doctor characteristic or practice factor was found to be associated with a successful outcome.

Factors reported by patients as helping or preventing reduction

Of the 31 patients who reported reduction of benzodiazepines over the trial period 25 (81%) said that they received support from their general practitioner which they found to be helpful (10 out of the 11 reducers in the control group and 15 out of the 20 in the intervention group). Six patients (19%) received helpful support from a friend or relative and three (10%) from another health professional. The 20 reducers in the intervention group had received the self-help booklet and of these 13 (65%) found it helpful. Three quarters of the doctors (18/24 of those with patients with booklets) also reported that the booklet was helpful in the everyday management of patients on benzodiazepines.

Fifty nine patients reported no reduction in their benzodiazepine consumption during the study. The commonest reason given for this was inability to sleep without the tablets (reported by 34 subjects). Twenty three patients thought they were better on the tablets, seven said they were too frightened to come off and two patients indicated that their doctor thought they were better off taking the tablets.

Continued →

Interviews with general practitioners

Thirty one general practitioners took part in the study and of these 27 were interviewed. Of the 27 doctors, 15 were men, the mean age was 45 years and the mean numbers of years in practice was 15. Six of the 11 practices in which these doctors worked had a counsellor or other specialist mental health professional doing sessional work.

The conditions most frequently treated with benzodiazepines by the doctors were, in order: acute insomnia, chronic insomnia, chronic anxiety, acute severe anxiety and acute back pain. Acute depression was the condition least likely to be treated with benzodiazepines. The two most common reasons for continuing to prescribe long-term benzodiazepines to patients were because the patient wished to remain on benzodiazepines and that it was too much of a struggle for the patient to come off the tablets.

No doctor was currently under threat of litigation with regard to their prescribing of benzodiazepines but three knew colleagues who were. Eighteen doctors were not at all concerned about litigation and nine were slightly concerned.

Discussion

In this study, chronic users of benzodiazepines who received from their general practitioners brief advice on withdrawal and a self-help booklet were found to have been prescribed lower doses of medication during follow up in significantly greater numbers than controls. In relation to self-report data, patients receiving minimal intervention also tended to report reduction and stopping of benzodiazepines more often than control group patients. These results were achieved in a population with high rates of past depression, anxiety, alcohol abuse and attempted suicide. The study also demonstrated that asking chronic users to withdraw from their medication was not associated with psychological harm or increased consultation with the general practitioner. This applied whether the patients reported reduction or not, indicating that it is safe to ask patients to withdraw from benzodiazepines, regardless of whether they are successful in the end or not. The intervention group as a whole (and its two sub-groups of benzodiazepine consumption reducers and non-reducers) were all experiencing more qualitative withdrawal symptoms at six months compared with baseline. However, general health questionnaire scores and consultation rates were unchanged, suggesting that the withdrawal symptoms did not cause undue distress to patients. It is also of interest that intervention patients who reported no reduction were experiencing withdrawal symptoms, implying that they too were trying to cut down their consumption of benzodiazepines.

The birth date method of allocation used in this study has been both criticized[13] and defended.[14] When doctors know the meaning of the allocation, the possibility that they might manipulate selection of subjects applies as much to a random allocation as to one dependent on date of birth. The birth date method is easy to understand and apply, especially for non-researchers. It is unobtrusive in comparison with other methods of randomization and so the doctor is less likely to be distracted from important nonverbal cues in the consultation. Furthermore, to our knowledge there is no inherent bias to the use of birth dates.[14]

It has been said that lowering benzodiazepine dosage may do more harm than good, in that the patient suffers more distress because of the reduced dose, yet does not have the benefit of coming off the medication.[15] The supporters of this view have usually considered stopping

Continued →

benzodiazepines as the only successful outcome. The present research contradicts this view. Intervention patients who reported reduction in their benzodiazepine intake showed a modest psychiatric improvement over the trial period as judged by the general health questionnaire. Although this group included nine subjects who reported stopping taking benzodiazepines there was no improvement in the psychiatric status of these stoppers. However, among the 11 patients who reported decreasing but not stopping benzodiazepines, there was improvement. Lowering benzodiazepine dosage is therefore valuable in its own right and should be encouraged, even if the patient is unable to cease intake completely.

Among night-time users, individuals receiving minimal intervention were significantly more likely than controls to reduce their medication, both according to self-report and prescribing records. Among daytime users, however, there was no difference between intervention patients and controls. It seems therefore that daytime users require more than minimal intervention to help them withdraw from benzodiazepines. This finding also lends further weight to the argument for a separate classification of daytime and night-time users.

A number of factors were found to be associated with a successful outcome in the trial. Being on an antidepressant at the end of the study was strongly predictive of a recorded reduction in benzodiazepine prescribing. One explanation could be drug substitution, that is, patients were being transferred from one psychotropic to another, the antidepressant being used as a hypnotic or anxiolytic instead of the benzodiazepine. Another possibility is that depression, which is common among these patients,[16] is being successfully treated, thereby reducing the need for other psychotropic drugs. The area is clearly complex, as illustrated by the finding that patients excluded by their general practitioner from the research, on the grounds that it might be harmful to them, were much more likely than study patients to be on an antidepressant at the end of the trial. Nevertheless, it would seem a rational policy to identify depression in chronic users and it may be that treating this with an antidepressant will assist withdrawal of benzodiazepines.

Taking a low baseline dose of benzodiazepines and a short acting preparation were both associated with a greater chance of reduction as reported by patients. The first of these findings has been noted before,[6] but is still surprising as one would expect that being on a higher initial dose would give more scope for reduction. Shorter acting preparations are generally thought to carry a greater risk of withdrawal symptoms and consequently it is often recommended that they be substituted by a long acting drug such as diazepam when withdrawal is being considered.[15] The results of this study suggest that it may be better to leave patients on their short acting preparations when a dose reduction is being attempted. The link between more physical illness and successfully stopping benzodiazepines is also an unexpected finding. One explanation is that these individuals only require their medication to overcome the psychological distress associated with physical illness and having recovered from, or adapted to the latter, they no longer have any real need for tablets.

No particular characteristic of doctors or their practices was identified as being important in helping chronic users to withdraw. However, 81% of patients who reported reducing their benzodiazepine consumption identified their doctor's support as being helpful during withdrawal. The self-help booklet also received a positive response from both patients and doctors.

Continued →

Some chronic users can successfully reduce their intake of benzodiazepines with a simple and practical intervention delivered by their general practitioner. The intervention does not cause psychological distress or increased consultation and this applies whether individuals are successful in reducing their intake or not.

References

1. Taylor D 1987 Current usage of benzodiazepines in Britain. In: Freeman H. Rue Y (eds). Benzodiazepines in current clinical practice. London: Royal Society of Medicine Services
2. Williams P 1987 Long-term benzodiazepine use in general practice. In: Freeman H. Rue Y (eds). Benzodiazepines in current clinical practice. London: Royal Society of Medicines Services
3. Committee on Safety of Medicines. Benzodiazepines, dependence and withdrawal symptoms. Current Problems 1988; 21
4. Committee on the Review of Medicines 1980 Systematic review of benzodiazepines. BMJ 280: 910–912
5. National Health Service Management Executive 1992 The health of the nation: first steps for the NHS. London: NHSME
6. Cormack M A, Owens R G, Dewey M E 1989 The effect of minimal interventions by general practitioners on long-term benzodiazepine use. J R Coll Gen Pract 39: 408–411
7. Cormack M A, Sweeney K G, Hughes-Jones H, Foot G A 1994 Evaluation of an easy, cost-effective strategy for cutting benzodiazepine use in general practice. Br J Gen Pract 44: 5–8
8. Ashworth M, King M B 1993 Benzodiazepine withdrawal among chronic daytime users in general practice. Psychiatr Bull 17: 77–78
9. Goldberg D P 1972 The detection of psychiatric disorder by questionnaire. Oxford University Press
10. Rodrigo E K, Williams P 1986 Frequency of self-reported 'anxiolytic withdrawal' symptoms in a group of female students experiencing anxiety. Psychol Med 16: 467–472
11. Machin D, Campbell M J 1987 Statistical tables for the design of clinical trials. Oxford: Blackwell Scientific
12. King M B 1994 Long-term benzodiazepine users – a mixed bag. Br J Addiction (in press)
13. Altman D G 1991 Randomisation. BMJ 302: 1481–1482.
14. King M B, Bashir K 1991 Randomisation [letter]. BMJ 303: 415
15. Russell J, Lader M 1992 (eds). Guidelines for the prevention and treatment of benzodiazepine dependence. London: Mental Health Foundation
16. Rodrigo E K, King M B, Williams P 1988 Health of long-term benzodiazepine users. BMJ 296: 603–606

Acknowledgements

We thank all the patients, doctors and practices who participated in the study. K B was supported by a grant from the Royal College of General Practitioners.

Address for correspondence

Dr K Bashir, Academic Department of Psychiatry, Royal Free Hospital School of Medicine, Pond Street, London NW3 2QG

CHAPTER 7

Can we improve our management of acute asthma?
An approach to using clinical guidelines

Chris Griffiths and Gene Feder

The clinical problem

The third patient in the morning surgery of an inner-city East London general practice is Mr Davies, a 50 year old council worker with asthma. He gives a 2-day history of increasing wheeze and shortness of breath. His usual medication is inhaled beclomethasone dipropionate, 800 mcg bd, with inhaled salbutamol as required. He has good inhaler technique and adheres well to his medication regimen. He is breathless but can complete sentences, has a respiratory rate of 20 breaths per minute and a pulse rate of 100 beats per minute. His peak expiratory flow rate (PEF) is 350 litres per minute with an expected PEF of 500 litres per minute. Whilst there are many important aspects to the management of acute asthma, the one addressed here is the question of when and how to use systemic rescue steroids.

You remember reading a recent review which surprised you by questioning the benefits of prescribing systemic rescue steroids in acute asthma (McFadden & Hejal 1995). When you discussed this at the time, a colleague pointed out that this article was not a systematic review, and reported neither a formal search strategy nor explicit methods of assessing research trials. In addition, your current practice, derived from your undergraduate medical education and junior doctor's experience, includes prescribing oral steroids in a tapering dose for at least 1 week. You decide to determine how valid a treatment the use of systemic steroids is, and to answer a range of related questions that might help you provide the most effective treatment for Mr Davies – and the several hundred other patients with acute asthma you will undoubtedly see during your career as a general practitioner.

You formulate the following questions about a 50-year-old adult, taking 800 mcg inhaled steroid per day, presenting in general practice with an acute exacerbation of asthma:

1. Are systemic steroids an effective (and cost-effective) treatment?
2. Is there a threshold of severity at which to begin rescue steroids?
3. What is the optimum dose of systemic steroids?
4. Should steroids be given intravenously or by mouth?
5. Does the dose need to be tapered?

Continued →

The clinical problem *(cont'd)*

6. How long should the course last?
7. Does prescribing steroids reduce the chances of admission to hospital?
8. What is the incidence of serious side-effects?

The priority is to treat Mr Davies immediately. This you do according to your usual practice (40 mg oral prednisolone daily, with a tapering dose to zero over the next week, 5 mg nebulized salbutamol, with advice about use of bronchodilator, use of PEF meter and written instructions on when to call for further assistance in the event of deterioration). You ask him to return the next day for review.

Introduction

Clinical guidelines have the potential to play a central role in bringing the results of research to the consultation (Sackett 1996). Guidelines are particularly relevant for general practitioners, who meet a much wider spectrum of clinical conditions than do hospital specialists. If guidelines are to be a tool for evidence-based practice they need to represent research evidence accurately; unfortunately this is often not the case. Some are developed by agencies with interests in promoting a particular product, and many provide little or no documentation about their development or the research on which their recommendations are based. These deficiencies make it difficult for users to assess potential bias in their content or to extrapolate recommendations to their patients. With these pitfalls in mind, general practitioners need to develop skills in finding relevant guidelines, distinguishing good guidelines from bad, and learning how to apply their recommendations in consultations.

What is a clinical guideline?

A generally accepted definition comes from Lohr & Field (1992): 'Guidelines are systematically developed statements to assist practitioner and patient decisions about appropriate care for specific clinical circumstances.'

This definition highlights three important features of contemporary guidelines. Firstly, they should be systematically developed, i.e. through a formal and explicit process that searches out the best evidence and applies it to the clinical question. This process needs to be described so that potential users of the guidelines can judge their quality. Secondly, guidelines should assist, but not inflexibly dictate, health care decisions; as Sackett has pointed out, evidence-based health care involves combining the best clinical evidence with individual clinical judgement (Sackett et al 1996). Thirdly, guidelines should address specific clinical questions. This helps ensure that guideline developers have a well-defined task and that guideline users are clear about the degree to which they can extrapolate recommendations to their patients.

The proliferation of clinical guidelines has brought two important challenges for those writing or commissioning these documents: firstly, how to develop guidelines that are scientifically 'valid', i.e. that accurately reflect the results of the best-quality research on which they are based; and secondly, how to ensure guidelines change practice. As clinicians trying to bring research evidence into our consultations, our challenges are different but relate to both of these: how to recognize a valid guideline, and then use the information therein to achieve the greatest cost-effective improvements in health for our patients.

Aims of this chapter

Our chapter addresses this challenge by taking an example commonly faced in general practice: the management of a patient with acute asthma.

Specifically, the aims of this chapter are:

1. to demonstrate how to define clinical questions
2. to discuss why one might look to clinical guidelines for answers (rather than other sources of evidence)
3. to demonstrate how to find relevant guidelines
4. to demonstrate both the advantages and limitations of using clinical guidelines
5. to provide advice on how one might use guidelines to develop a practice policy.

How to access useful research evidence

There are at least five ways of trying to answer the questions you have formulated. Firstly, you might ask a respected colleague, but realize their answer may be based on the same

Table 7.1 Relative merits of different sources of evidence

Source of advice	Advantages	Disadvantages
Ask a respected colleague	Convenient Fast Sociable	Uncertain relationship to the evidence
Run own MEDLINE search and appraise article(s)	Comprehensive search Access to complete data	Slow – may need to retrieve and appraise several articles
Hand (or CD-ROM) search of ACP/EBM* journal summaries of high-quality articles	Convenient Fast	Only covers recent papers Summaries only
CD-ROM search of COCHRANE LIBRARY summaries	Convenient Fast	Only covers recent papers Summaries only Cochrane not yet reported on asthma
Relevant clinical guidelines	Fast Potentially comprehensive summaries of large bodies of evidence	Quality of guidelines vary May be out of date Summaries only

American College of Physicians and *Evidence-based Medicine* journals. These are available as 'Best Evidence' on CD-ROM.

received wisdom you are questioning. Other approaches to accessing useful research evidence are recommended in an *Evidence-based Medicine* note (Sackett 1996): you could run your own MEDLINE search to find a relevant article and critically appraise this; you could search (by hand or by CD-ROM) the summaries of high-quality studies in the journal *Evidence-based Medicine*; similarly, you could search the COCHRANE LIBRARY reports on CD-ROM. Lastly, you could try to answer these questions by looking at guidelines for asthma management. The advantages and disadvantages of these strategies are set out in Table 7.1.

Since guidelines potentially offer the fastest and most convenient way of both accessing a high-quality systematic review of a large body of research literature and getting specific clinical recommendations, you decide to pursue this option.

How to access useful guidelines on asthma

Three asthma guidelines are readily available to you: the

Table 7.2 Useful Web site addresses

---

1. **http://www.ohsu.edu/bicc-informatics/ebm/ebm_topics.htm**
The searchable database is currently available only within the Oregon Health Sciences University network. However, a list of documents included in the database indexed by Medical Subject Heading (MeSH) terms is available here.
All documents on this list show evidence of a literature search to identify high-quality evidence on the topic or include a critical appraisal of a single article. The list has been divided into several sublists to facilitate downloading. To locate a specific MeSH term, select the correct sublist below and then use your browser's find button and enter the term to search for.
2. **http://text.nlm.nih.gov**
The National Library of Medicine's Web site with access to all the Agency for Health Care Policy and Research guidelines, National Institutes for Health consensus statements and health technology assessments.
3. **http://www.shef.ac.uk/~scharr/ir/netting.html**
Produced by the dynamic Andrew Booth at Sheffield's School of Health and Related Research. 'A virtual core library for evidence-based practice', with links to many sites relevant to guideline developers and adaptors.

British Thoracic Society (BTS) asthma guidelines (British Asthma Guidelines Co-ordinating Committee 1997), the local East London asthma guidelines (East London Clinical Guidelines Project 1996), and the North of England (NoE) evidence-based guidelines (North of England Evidence-based Guidelines Development Group 1996) published by the *British Medical Journal* both on paper and on the Internet. A more comprehensive way of searching for guidelines covering a particular topic is by accessing guidelines listings on relevant Web sites (see Table 7.2).

Choosing the best-quality guidelines

In trying to find the most reliable answers to your questions, your first task is to choose the most valid (i.e. least biased) guidelines. The most important question to answer when assessing the validity of guidelines is: was evidence systematically collected, critically appraised, graded for strength, and linked to specific recommendations?

The British Thoracic Society and the local East London asthma guidelines are readily available on your surgery bookshelf. The latter state that they are a local adaptation of the systematic review of published asthma literature carried out by the NoE development group, and give the Internet reference to the NoE guidelines themselves (http://www.tecc.co.uk/bmj/asthma/ast01.htm). On the main practice computer it takes less than 5 minutes to key in the reference, find the relevant section on oral steroid

Table 7.3 Criteria for high-quality clinical guidelines

Criterion	British Thoracic Society asthma guidelines	East London asthma guidelines	North of England asthma guidelines
Systematic literature search	No	Yes	Yes
Explicit linkage of graded evidence to recommendations	No	Yes	Yes

prescribing and print it out. An alternative is to find the paper version of these guidelines in the practice library (North of England Evidence-based Guidelines Development Group 1996). Looking at the three guidelines you compare the methods used to develop and present them. The NoE Guidelines Development Group report using a systematic search strategy, followed by grading of evidence from individual papers identified, and subsequent derivation of recommendations explicitly linked to the quality of the evidence. By contrast, the BTS guidelines used an expert panel to write discussion papers which were then used as a basis for developing recommendations at a consensus conference. The East London guidelines were based on the NoE systematic review with adaptation to local circumstances. All three development groups contained representatives from key relevant disciplines.

It seems clear from the assessment shown in Table 7.3 that your 'best bets' are the East London and the North of England guidelines. Since the latter is a source of the local document, you decide to make this your first choice.

A more detailed appraisal of guidelines quality can be carried out with a validated appraisal tool (Cluzeau et al 1997).

Grading of research evidence and derivation of recommendations

The North of England Guidelines Development Group searched MEDLINE and BATH INFORMATION AND DATA SERVICES (BIDS) databases for 1985–94 for published studies of asthma diagnosis and treatment, which were then assessed for methodological rigour and clinical relevance (Eccles et al 1996). Studies were categorized according to study design:

I. based on well-designed, randomized controlled trials, meta-analyses, or systematic reviews

II.   based on well-designed cohort or case control studies
III. based on uncontrolled studies or consensus.

Note: Meta-analysis is a technique that quantitatively combines the results of systematically identified studies addressing a defined question to produce an overview describing an effect size with confidence intervals – see Chapter 9.

The development group qualitatively summarized the content of identified research to give a set of agreed statements. Recommendations were then derived by informal consensus and graded by strength of evidence and importance for practice. The relationships between categories of evidence and strength of recommendations are as follows:

A.   directly based on category I evidence
B.   directly based on category II evidence or extrapolated recommendation from category I evidence
C.   directly based on category III evidence or extrapolated recommendation from category I or II evidence.

Interpreting and using guidelines or recommendations

The text under the heading 'oral steroids' in the NoE guidelines is reprinted at the end of this chapter. In summary, the guidelines recommend:

1. early use of systemic steroids for acute asthma
2. use of the oral in preference to intravenous route
3. no need to taper the dose for courses of up to 2 weeks.

Additional conclusions are:

1. Systemic steroids reduce the likelihood of admission to hospital.
2. 'Medium' and 'high' doses may be superior to 'low' doses.
3. Systemic steroids are a safe treatment but should be avoided in patients with a history of gastrointestinal bleeding or taking anticoagulants.

The interpretation of these recommendations depends not only on the overall validity of the guidelines, but on the applicability of the trials on which the recommendations are based to Mr Davies. There are a number of guides to interpreting guidelines and their recommendations

Table 7.4 Using clinical practice guidelines

---

a. **Are the recommendations in this guideline valid?**
    Primary guide
    - Was the evidence systematically collected, critically appraised and graded and linked to specific recommendations?

    Secondary guide
    - Were all important decision options and outcomes clearly specified?
    - Are the relative preferences that key stakeholders attach to the outcomes of decisions (including benefits, risks and costs) identified and explicitly considered?
    - Is the guideline resistant to clinically sensible variations in practice?

b. **Is this valid guideline potentially useful? Does the guideline offer an opportunity for significant improvement in the quality of care?**
    - Is there a large variation in current practice?
    - Does the guideline contain new evidence (or old evidence not yet acted upon) that could have an important impact on management?
    - Would the guideline affect the management of so many people, or concern individuals at such high risk, or involve such high costs that even small changes in practice could have major impacts on health outcomes or resources?
    - How large, and how precise, is the treatment effect?
    - Can the guideline strategy help you in managing your patient?

(After Sackett et al 1997)

(Hayward et al 1995, Wilson et al 1995, Cluzeau et al 1997, Sackett et al 1997). From these sources we provide a number of key questions (see Table 7.4).

a. Are the recommendations in this guideline valid?

Primary guide

i. Was evidence systematically collected, critically appraised and graded and linked to specific recommendations?
This is addressed above.

Secondary guides

i. Were all important decision options and outcomes clearly specified?
In Mr Davies's case the main treatment options are to treat with steroids (intravenous or oral), or to increase the dose of inhaled steroids or bronchodilator to a maximum. Out of these, the NoE guideline only seems to have explicitly considered the use of systemic steroids as the treatment option. It is not clear whether the development group considered alternatives. The important patient outcomes in this case are improved lung function, prevention of admission to hospital, prevention of relapse, and prevention

of unwanted side-effects. All these outcomes are addressed by the guidelines.

ii. Are the relative preferences that key stakeholders attach to the outcomes of decisions (including benefits, risks and costs) identified and explicitly considered?
This question can be answered on two levels: either at the level of guideline development or of guideline implementation.

In the development of guidelines, the relative preferences of stakeholders about outcomes will depend on their reason(s) for developing the guidelines. The most important outcome for a pharmaceutical company might be increased use of their product; that for an American health maintenance organization might be cost containment; for a British health authority it might be overall cost-effectiveness. Stakeholders in guideline development should be explicit about sources of funding, and the composition of the development group. In the case of the NoE guideline, whilst we have no details of relative preferences that the developers attached to different outcomes, the source of funding was a health authority and the development group comprised a range of relevant clinicians (e.g. chest consultants, general practitioners, practice nurses). One could speculate that the developers' overall outcome preference in this case was cost-effective health care, but this is neither identified nor explicitly considered.

At the level of implementation, the key stakeholders are yourself and Mr Davies. Guidelines can incorporate relative preferences at this level either qualitatively (Rabeneck et al 1997) or quantitatively, assuming adequate information is available, as a clinical guidance decision tree (Dowie 1997). The latter allows the insertion of utilities that the patient or you yourself attach to different outcomes (e.g. admission to hospital, risk of side-effects of medication, relapse etc.). In the absence of this information, incorporation of relative preferences is limited to you and your patient's interpretation of potential benefits and harms. Costs are not addressed, although the cost of the steroid treatment itself is minimal.

iii. Is the guideline resistant to clinically sensible variations in practice?
The introduction to the NoE guidelines states that the recommendations are given as guidance, acknowledging the

need for flexibility in their application depending on clinical circumstances. A sensible variation in practice might be the avoidance of oral steroids in a patient with a recent history of a bleeding duodenal ulcer.

b. Is this valid guideline potentially useful? Does the guideline offer an opportunity for significant improvement in the quality of care?

i. Is there a large variation in current practice?
Numerous reports attest to the numbers of patients who are admitted to hospital with acute asthma without having begun systemic steroids (e.g. Blainey et al 1991). In addition, discussion amongst your colleagues reveals uncertainty over the need to taper doses.

ii. Does the guideline contain new evidence (or old evidence not yet acted upon) that could have an important impact on management?
The guidelines contain important old evidence not yet acted upon.

iii. Would the guideline affect the management of so many people, or concern individuals at such high risk, or involve such high costs that even small changes in practice could have major impacts on health outcomes or resources?
You remember a recent report highlighting that East London has one of the highest rates of hospital admissions for asthma in the country, and that asthma admissions cost the local health authority around a million pounds per year (Griffiths et al 1997). The potential outcome and resource impact of increasing steroid prescribing in acute exacerbations would be positive.

iv. How large, and how precise, is the treatment effect?
In the case of the effect of systemic steroid use on admission to hospital, the NoE guidelines gave treatment effects as odds ratios: 'Use of steroids early in the treatment of exacerbations reduces subsequent admissions in adults: Odds ratio 0.47 (95% CI 0.27–0.79).'

The odds ratio is a measure of relative risk. It gives the odds of an event occurring in a treatment group, divided by the odds of it occurring in a control group. If the odds are the same in the two groups, their ratio will be 1. Thus, the best estimate of the chance of admission to hospital in patients treated with steroid is roughly half that of those not treated. The confidence intervals of this estimate indicate that the true value has a 95% chance of lying somewhere between 0.27 and 0.79.

Odds ratios and relative risks give no information about the underlying risk of the event. For instance, they do not allow you to distinguish between a 50% reduction in a small (and perhaps clinically irrelevant) baseline risk and a large and important baseline risk. The reduction in absolute risk of admission would be a more useful guide; this depends on the proportion of patients with exacerbations admitted to hospital with asthma locally. The local East London guidelines provide this information, giving the numbers needed to treat (NNT) to prevent one admission to hospital, a measure of absolute risk. This illustrates an advantage of local guidelines in that they can provide information in a local context. The NNT is the reciprocal of the absolute risk reduction. Roughly 2 in 10 patients seen in East London accident and emergency departments (AEDs) with acute asthma are admitted. Thus the NNT with oral steroids is about 11 patients; this represents a good basis for using oral steroids in AEDs. Assuming that for general practice the proportion of patients admitted to hospital with acute asthma were about 1 in 20, the NNT would be 36 patients. The average general practitioner will see about 30 patients with asthma exacerbations per year (Neville et al 1992); a 10-day course of 40 mg prednisolone per day costs about 75 pence (British National Formulary 1997). Thus, this represents a good *and* cost-effective treatment option.

Odds ratios and event rates can be most easily converted to NNTs using Table 7.5. (See also Sackett et al 1997, Bandolier 1997.). Odds ratios (ORs) are given along the top line; control event rates (CERs) are given down the left-hand side. NNTs are found by reading off where the OR column and the CER row intersect. For instance, if the CER (in our case, the proportion of patients admitted with acute asthma via local AEDs) is 2 in 10 or 0.2, and the OR for the effect of oral steroids is roughly 0.5 (actually 0.47), the NNT is 11 patients.

v. Can the guideline strategy help you in managing Mr Davies?
The above discussion suggests that the answer here is yes. However, a crucial question remains: to what degree can the results of this research (and therefore the guidelines' recommendations) be extrapolated to your clinical situation? The answer to this depends on the internal and external validity of the meta-analysis.

Table 7.5 Conversion of odds ratios and event rates into numbers needed to treat (NNT) (after Bandolier 1997)

Control event rate	Odds ratios								
	0.5	0.55	0.6	0.65	0.7	0.75	0.8	0.85	0.9
0.05	41	46	52	59	69	83	104	139	209
0.1	21	24	27	31	36	43	54	73	110
0.2	11	13	14	17	20	24	30	40	61
0.3	8	9	10	12	14	18	22	30	46
0.4	7	8	9	10	12	15	19	26	40
0.5	6	7	8	9	11	14	18	25	38
0.7	6	7	9	10	13	16	20	28	44
0.9	12	15	18	22	27	34	46	64	101

Internal validity of the meta-analysis. The internal validity of the meta-analysis refers to the methodological quality of the original studies. If these (or the meta-analysis summarizing them) are of poor quality, the results may be unreliable and the authors may be drawing unjustified conclusions. Potential problems here may be *publication bias*, where studies showing no benefit of steroid use fail to get published and so cannot contribute to the meta-analysis, or *poor statistical technique* by the authors, such that conclusions are unreliable. Unless you search out the original meta-analysis, you are entirely reliant on the quality of the guideline development group process. However, the NoE Guidelines Development Group's method for selection of evidence makes the inclusion of poor-quality studies less likely.

External validity of the meta-analysis This refers to the extent to which the patients and their clinical circumstances are similar to your own patients and their circumstances. For instance, 73% of the papers contributing to this meta-analysis came from the USA; 67% of the papers addressed patients admitted to hospital. Was the severity of asthma similar to that seen in routine British general practice? Again, unless you return to the original meta-analysis you are reliant on the guidelines development group's competence and opinions on extrapolation. In fact, all studies included in the analysis defined exacerbations of asthma as 'patients who had experienced increased symptoms, reduced pulmonary function as measured by FEV_1, or an increased use of bronchodilators prior to arrival in the emergency department'. Whilst no objective thresholds for starting treatment are given (for instance, as

percentage reduction in PEFR), Mr Davies fits these
qualitative inclusion criteria.

Relative preferences and cost-effectiveness
The guidelines give no information on how individual
preferences of the patient or clinician might be incorporated,
or how these might affect the outcome of care, and no
details of relative cost-effectiveness of different treatment
options. These omissions are common even in otherwise
good-quality guidelines, mostly because the underlying
data are not available

Other unanswered questions
You still lack answers to two of your original questions.
What dose of steroid is effective, and how long should the
course last? The NoE guideline comments that 'medium and
high' doses were more effective than 'low' doses. These are
not defined (although the original meta-analysis defines
'low' as less than 30 mg of prednisolone every 6 hours, i.e.
less than 120 mg per day). Although further research needs
to be done on steroid dosage, this could suggest that many
steroid courses are of inadequate dose, particularly if they
are tapered. The NoE guidelines make a consensus (grade
C) recommendation that '30–40 mg prednisolone be given
until the episode has resolved, symptoms are controlled,

Reviewing Mr Davies

Mr Davies returns the next morning. On the basis of your critical review of
available guidelines you not only feel more confident in some aspects of
management, but also are more aware of the limitations of available research and
its incorporation into clinical guidelines. You are able to suggest adjustments to
Mr Davies's treatment and to reassure him with additional information.

- Adjustments to his treatment:
  — You ask him to continue his dose rather than to taper it.
- Additional information for Mr Davies:
  — The steroid treatment has a good chance of preventing his admission to
    hospital.
  — You were justified in suggesting he take the steroids by mouth.
  — The treatment has a low chance of serious gastrointestinal side-effects.
  You are also alert to new studies which address your unanswered questions:
- What is the most appropriate dose of prednisolone?
- What is the optimum duration of treatment?

and lung function values have returned to previous best. Although 7 days' treatment will often be sufficient, treatment may be needed for up to 21 days.'

Using clinical guidelines to develop a practice policy

There are two additional means by which clinical guidelines can bring useful evidence to your practice: firstly, by developing a practice policy derived from valid guidelines, and secondly, by generating evidence-based audit standards (Baker & Fraser 1995).

Given the uncertainty and variation in use of systemic steroids amongst your practice colleagues in patients with acute asthma, it would be a useful next step to arrange to review your practice policy towards management of acute asthma. Grimshaw & Russell (1993) showed in their systematic review of the efficacy of guidelines that guidelines were most likely to change practice if they were developed by the clinicians who were ultimately to use them, were introduced via a specific educational intervention (such as a discussion meeting), and were implemented via prompts to clinicians during consultations. Developing a practice policy through a clinical meeting where the guidelines you have reviewed are discussed might increase the chances of practice members following the policy recommendations. The growing role of nurses in asthma management requires their involvement in practice policy, and guidelines, like audit, provide a sound multidisciplinary focus. One of the simplest and most powerful ways to implement policies or guidelines recommendations within a practice is to develop and use computer templates or notes prompts for use during consultations with patients (Feder et al 1995).

Secondly, the availability of valid guidelines provides the opportunity for the practice to agree and set evidence-based audit standards. In the case of oral steroid use, this standard might be that oral steroids will have been prescribed, without tapering, in all patients presenting with acute severe asthma (comprising increased symptoms, reduced pulmonary function, or an increased use of bronchodilators), with the exception of patients with gastrointestinal bleeding, those on oral anticoagulants, or those who decline. Whilst audit and feedback in themselves are relatively weak in changing clinician behaviour (Davis et al 1995), combination with other strategies (such as computer templates) can make them more effective.

References

Baker R, Fraser R C 1995 Development of review criteria: linking guidelines and assessment of quality. British Medical Journal 311: 370–373

Bandolier 1997 Calculating NNTs. Bandolier 36: 2

Blainey D, Lomas D, Beale A, Partridge M 1991 The cost of acute asthma – how much is preventable? Health Trends 22: 151–153

British National Formulary 1997 British Medical Association and the Royal Pharmaceutical Society of Great Britain, London

British Asthma Guidelines Co-ordinating Committee 1997 British Guidelines on asthma management: 1995 review and position statement 1997. Thorax 52: S1–24

Carson J L, Strom B L, Schinnar R, Duff A, Sim E 1991 The low risk of upper gastrointestinal bleeding in patients dispensed corticosteroids. American Journal of Medicine 91: 223–228

Cluzeau F, Littlejohns P, Grimshaw J, Feder G 1997 Appraisal instrument for clinical guidelines. Version I. St George's Hospital Medical School

Davis D A, Thompson M A, Oxman A D, Haynes R B 1995 Changing physician performance: a systematic review of the effect of continuing medical education strategies. Journal of the American Medical Association 274: 700–705

Dowie J 1997 Alternative approaches to clinical guidance: guideline statements and clinical guidance trees. Paper presented at workshop 'From evidence to recommendations: exploring the methods', NHS Centre for Reviews and Dissemination, University of York

East London Clinical Guidelines Project 1996 Adult asthma general practice guidelines. Department of General Practice and Primary Care, St Bartholomew's and the Royal London Hospitals, London

Eccles M, Clapp Z, Grimshaw J, Adams P C, Higgins B, Purves I, Russell I 1996 North of England evidence-based guidelines development project: methods of guideline development. British Medical Journal 312: 760–762

Feder G, Griffiths C, Highton C, Eldridge S, Spence M, Southgate L 1995 Do clinical guidelines introduced with practice based education improve care of asthmatic and diabetic patients? A randomised controlled trial in general practices in east London. British Medical Journal 311: 1473–1478

Griffiths C J, Sturdy P, Naish J, Omar R, Dolan S, Feder G 1997 Hospital admissions for asthma in East London: associations with characteristics of local general practices, prescribing and population. British Medical Journal 314: 482–486

Grimshaw J M, Russell I T 1993 Effect of clinical guidelines on medical practice: a systematic review of rigorous evaluations. Lancet 342: 1317–1322

Hayward R S, Wilson M C, Tunis S R, Bass E B, Guyatt G 1995 Users' guides to the medical literature VIII. How to use clinical practice guidelines. A Are the recommendations valid? Journal of the American Medical Association 274: 570–574

Lohr K N, Field M J 1992 Guidelines for clinical practice: from development to use. National Academy Press, Washington DC

McFadden E R, Hejal R 1995 Asthma. Lancet 345: 1215–1220

Neville R, Clark R, Hoskins G, Smith B for General Practitioners in Asthma Group 1992 National asthma attack audit. British Medical Journal 306: 559–562

North of England Evidence-based Guidelines Development Group 1996 Summary version of evidence-based guidelines for the primary care management of asthma in adults. British Medical Journal 312: 762–766

North of England Study of Standards and Performance in General Practice 1992 Medical audit in general practice: effect on doctors' clinical behaviour and the health of patients with common childhood conditions. British Medical Journal 304: 1480–1488

Rabeneck L, McCullough L B, Wray N P 1997 Ethically justified, clinically comprehensive guidelines for percutaneous endoscopic gastrotomy tube placement. Lancet 349: 496–498

Rowe B H, Keller J L, Oxman D A 1992 Effectiveness of steroid therapy in acute exacerbations of asthma: a meta-analysis. American Journal of Emergency Medicine 10: 301–310

Sackett D L 1996 On the need for evidence-based medicine (EBM Note). Evidence-based Medicine 1: 5–6

Sackett D L, Richardson W S, Rosenberg W, Haynes R B 1997 Evidence-based medicine: how to practise and teach EBM. Churchill Livingstone, London

Sackett D L, Rosenberg W M, Gray J A, Richardson W S 1996 Evidence-based medicine: what it is and what it isn't. British Medical Journal 312: 71–72

Wilson M C, Hayward R S, Tunis S R, Bass E B, Guyatt G 1995 Users' guides to the medical literature VIII. How to use clinical practice guidelines. B What are the recommendations and will they help you in caring for your patients? Journal of the American Medical Association 274: 1630–1632

North of England asthma guidelines recommendations on the use of oral steroids in acute asthma

Oral Steroids

Recommendations

- Steroids should be used in exacerbations of asthma (grade A)
- They should be given orally as intravenous administration offers no advantages (grade A)
- When used in short courses of up to 2 weeks the dose of oral steroids does not need to be tapered; they can be stopped from full dosages (grade C)

Statement

Steroid therapy provides important benefits to patients presenting with acute exacerbations of asthma; oral and intravenous dosing are equally effective (level I).

From meta-analysis of 30 relevant randomized controlled trials looking at the effectiveness of steroid therapy in acute exacerbations of asthma Rowe et al (1992) concluded that: the use of steroids early in the treatments of asthmatic exacerbations reduces subsequent admissions in adults (odds ratio 0.47: 95% confidence interval 0.27, 0.97); steroids are effective in preventing relapse in the outpatient treatment of asthmatic exacerbations (odds ratio 0.15: 95% CI 0.05, 0.44); and oral and intravenous steroids appear to have equivalent effects on pulmonary function in acute exacerbation (effects size –0.07; 95% CI–0.39, 0.25). They could not produce any summary conclusions about dose and dosing, though 'low' doses were not as effective as 'medium and high doses'.

Reference

Rowe B H, Keller J L, Oxmand D A 1992 Effectiveness of steroid therapy in acute exacerbations of asthma: a meta-analysis. American Journal of Emergency Medicine 10: 301–310

Statement

Used in short courses oral steroids are safe; they produce very low rates of gastrointestinal bleeding. The greatest risk is in those with a past history of gastrointestinal bleeding or taking anticoagulants (level III).

Carson et al (1991) reported a descriptive analysis of the records of 90 880 patients who received oral steroids (for dermatitis as well as asthma). They show a very low incidence of gastrointestinal bleeding and conclude that prophylaxis against bleeding is not generally necessary. In subgroup analysis the biggest risk was in people who had upper GI bleeding in the past and in subjects also taking oral anticoagulants, but even here the incidence was low.

Comment

The *British National Formulary* states that: 'corticosteriod therapy is weakly linked with peptic ulceration; the use of soluble or enteric coated preparations to reduce risk is speculative only.'

Reference

Carson J L, Strom B L, Schinnar R, Duff A and Sim E 1991 The low risk of upper gastrointestinal bleeding in patients dispensed corticosteriods. American Journal of Medicine 91: 223–228

CHAPTER 8

How can we check the quality of our diabetic care?
An approach to clinical audit

Mayur Lakhani and Richard Baker

The clinical problem

Dr Y is a GP registrar attached to one of us (ML) at a three-doctor inner-city practice with a list size of 6000. Dr Y was contemplating undertaking an audit of diabetes care at the practice as part of summative assessment. We run a diabetic clinic and there are 90 diabetics on the practice diabetic register. We had a meeting to plan the audit and ask ourselves a number of questions, but our main preoccupation was to conduct an effective, worthwhile audit. For us the key issue was to identify the 'gold standard' criteria against which to judge the care that we give to our diabetics. Dr Y gathered a number of papers and documents to help us plan our audit. We had also been sent several audit packages from our local primary care audit group (formally, medical audit advisory group or MAAG), and an example of an actual audit done by another practice with the consent of the GP at that practice, Dr K. In the first instance we looked at Dr K's audit (see Table 8.2, p. 142).

Introduction

In this chapter we shall first briefly consider what we mean by evidence-based audit, and then illustrate critical appraisal of audit reports, published multipractice audits and audit guidelines by reference to diabetes in primary care.

Most general practitioners (GPs) have had some experience of audit. The number of practices participating in audit has increased from 57% in 1991/2 to 86% in 1993/4, with many practices having completed a full audit (Baker et al 1995). The General Medical Council (GMC) document, 'Duties of a doctor', states that a doctor 'should take part in regular and systematic audit' (GMC 1995). GPs may meet audit or be asked to make decisions relating to audit in a number of situations. A GP may decide to undertake an

Table 8.1 Steps in systematic audit (Fraser et al 1998)

- Select topic.
- Identify specific aims.
- Agree target criteria and standards.
- Devise method of data collection.
- Collect data.
- Analyse and compare with target criteria and standards.
- Agree and implement changes.
- Collect further data to evaluate change.

audit, in which case one question that may arise is, 'How is a topic to be selected?' A practice may be asked to take part in a multipractice audit organized by their local primary care audit group, in which several practices undertake the same audit. In this case, the doctor might reasonably ask, 'Are the criteria valid?' and 'Is this a sound audit project?' A GP registrar may wish to undertake an audit because an audit project is now a compulsory component of summative assessment for GP registrars. Within the chronic disease management programme, regular audit of asthma and diabetes is expected and these are popular topics for audit.

Many organizations produce 'audit packages', and there may be several audit protocols on a single clinical topic. How can a doctor choose from amongst them? Many audits are now also published and therefore GPs need to be able to appraise an audit publication critically, adopting a structured approach to critical appraisal (Bhopal & Thomson 1991). For these reasons and many more, general practitioners need to be able to develop and use an evidence-based approach to managing clinical audit in their practices, that should include an ability to appraise an audit report and/or an audit tool.

An evidence-based approach to audit

Systematic audit is a cycle or spiral which consists of a series of particular steps (Fraser et al 1998) (see Table 8.1). An audit project begins with the need to select a topic, followed by the formulation of explicit aims and the identification of explicit criteria against which to judge performance. Actual performance must be determined by collection of objective data. Discrepancies between actual and desired performance then need to be addressed by selected strategies which may include feedback, facilitation or reminders. Data are then collected again to determine the extent to which appropriate changes have been made.

Measurement of performance

In measuring performance, explicit statements are needed about what to measure (i.e. the audit criteria) and what level of performance is expected (i.e. the standard). Criteria and standards are often confused. Criteria have been defined as: 'systematically developed statements that can be used to assess the appropriateness of health care decisions, services and outcomes' (Institute of Medicine 1992). On the other hand, a standard is: 'the percentage of events that should comply with the criterion' (Baker & Fraser 1995).

If measurements of actual performance in an audit are to be meaningful and of practical value, it is of fundamental importance that the audit criteria against which actual performance is to be judged are developed in compliance with the following key principles (Baker & Fraser 1995). Audit criteria must be:

- based on evidence
- prioritized
- measurable
- appropriate to the setting.

Since audit review criteria are the 'gold standard' against which performance is to be judged, it is of overriding importance that they must be credible. To achieve this status, they must be based on the best available current research evidence. Some elements of care are supported by more convincing evidence than others. In assessing performance it would be inappropriate to place the same weight on criteria that are supported only by moderate evidence as those supported by strong evidence. For these reasons audit criteria need to be prioritized according to the strength of evidence. The impact on outcome should also be taken into account. Audit criteria must be capable of being measured, and the wording must be sufficiently explicit to minimize opportunities for misunderstanding. This also ensures that multiple participants in an audit measure the same thing. Audit criteria must be appropriate to the setting in which they are to be used. For example, patients attending hospital outpatients departments are a selected group in comparison with those attending their general practitioner. Accordingly, patients with hypertension who are referred to hospitals are more likely to have secondary causes for their condition and a wide range of investigations may be warranted. However, such investigations, which are properly indicated in a hospital population, are much less likely to be appropriate for hypertensive patients attending their general practitioner.

Critical appraisal of an audit

Dr K is a GP in a rural practice of five doctors. His diabetes audit report consisted of the set of results shown in Table 8.2. We were quite interested in this audit with a view to replicating it, but first we wanted to be sure that it was a 'good' audit without any major flaws. We had no clear way of appraising the quality of this audit and so could not decide whether to duplicate it in our own practice. Our primary care audit group had given us two review tools which could help us to appraise the audit (Bhopal & Thomson 1991, Joint Audit Review Group 1995). Both these tools consist of a structured form to assess the quality of an audit report. They are both very similar but we decided to make use of the Lilly Audit Centre appraisal tool because it appeared slightly easier to use (see Table 8.3).

Looking at Dr K's audit we felt that there was insufficient information in the report to be able to judge the quality of the audit, so we decided to visit and interview him using the audit review tool as a guide. When we asked Dr K about the reason for undertaking the audit, he replied that this was expected under the chronic disease management

Table 8.2 Audit of 50 diabetics at Dr K's practice: proportion of patients with information recorded over the last 12 months (%)

Information	% patients
Weight recorded	60%
Blood pressure	80%
Glycated haemoglobin	60%
Lipids	40%
Family history	70%
Diet check	50%
Smoking	60%
Alcohol	30%
Feet	30%
Neuropathy	30%
Injection sites	45%
Diet checked	50%
Urea and electrolytes/creatinine	40%
Leaflets/education	40%

Table 8.3 Critical appraisal of an audit (Joint Audit Review Group 1995)

1. Reason for undertaking the audit:
   — A clear statement about why the audit was undertaken
2. Funding / conflict of interest:
   — What was the source of funding and does the audit promote any commercial product?
3. Planning of audit:
   — Was the planning of the audit multidisciplinary?
4. How were criteria selected?
   — No explicit criteria
   — National guideline
   — Local guideline
   — Literature review
   — Consultation with experts
   — Consultation with patients
5. Data collection:
   — Source of data
   — Clear instructions about which patients to include
   — Method of data collection
   — Sampling procedure
   — Sample size adequate
   — Data analysis
   — Verification / reliability of data
6. Results:
   — Were any deficiencies in care shown?
   — Was a second data collection completed?
7. Change:
   — What changes were recommended and how were they implemented? e.g. feedback, or educational intervention or other
8. Conclusions:
   — Benefits arising from the audit: patient, professional, service, other
   — Difficulties encountered in the audit
   — Was a second cycle completed and had an improvement taken place?

programme and he wanted to show that he was 'doing some audit'. The audit had not been funded or sponsored. When we asked him how he had planned the audit, Dr K stated that he planned the audit himself and selected the criteria according to what he thought constituted good care. This was based on their practice protocol, which was a modified version of a local health authority protocol.

Next, we asked how patients were selected. Dr K replied that the practice nurse was asked to choose 50 diabetic patients from the computer register but could not say if they had been randomly selected. He could not say how diabetes was defined, nor could he say why 50, when there were over 150 diabetics on the register. No advice had been taken about sample size. Children were excluded, but the cut-off age was not defined. As for data collection, Dr K had designed a form which the practice nurse had used to collect information. We asked if the data collected were verified by another person. This had not been done. Dr K was asked what was done if information was missing or not recorded in the notes. He did not have a policy to deal with this. As for the results, Dr K was generally pleased with the findings but thought that things could be improved. There were no obvious plans to make any changes or re-audit.

We felt that there were a number of question marks over Dr K's audit and we did not feel sufficiently confident to adopt it as the model for our own. In particular, we were not sure whether some of the criteria used were valid: for example, recording family history and measuring renal function routinely.

Critical appraisal of a paper on audit

We decided to look at the other materials provided by our local primary care audit group. Amongst the audit packages we had received, we were puzzled by the wide variety of criteria suggested in different ones. We wondered where the criteria came from and why there should be such a variation. Having read the documents, Dr Y generated a list of criteria which he would like to include in the audit (see Table 8.4).

ML felt overwhelmed by the list, which seemed to have far too many criteria. He was emphatic that the number of criteria should be reduced to make the audit more manageable, and although Dr Y agreed, we could not decide which ones were more important than others. We noticed that the methods used to choose criteria varied between different packages. Some did not have references to original research

Table 8.4 Dr Y's suggested criteria for a diabetes audit

- Retina examination
- Blood pressure check
- Random blood glucose measurements
- Urine testing
- Measurement of glycated haemoglobin
- Family history documented
- Dietary assessment
- Assessment of feet
- Urea and electrolytes and creatinine done
- Assessment for neuropathy
- Assessment of self-monitoring of urine/blood sugars
- Inspection of injection sites
- Regular weighing
- Assessment of symptoms
- Lipids checked
- Test for microalbuminuria
- Assessment of patient education

but others did, whilst some relied on recommendations by consultants. Some placed particular emphasis on investigations. In addition, there appeared to be a mixture of structure, process and outcome measures in the documents.

We decided to resolve this confusion by taking matters into our own hands and seeking additional information. The question we wanted to answer was: Which are valid criteria that should be included in an audit of diabetes in primary care? During our next visit to the local postgraduate education centre to attend a postgraduate meeting, we dropped in at the local library. We only had a few minutes before heading back to the practice, and with the help of the librarian we tried the simplest of searches using the terms 'diabetes', 'medical audit' and 'family practice' on MEDLINE (1992–7). Three articles appeared relevant: Dunn & Bough (1996); Benett et al (1994); Tunbridge et al (1993). We printed the abstracts and arranged for the full papers to be sent on. Dunn & Bough (1996) described the standards of care of 3974 diabetic patients in 37 practices in Poole, Dorset. Benett et al (1994) described emerging standards for diabetes care from a city-wide audit in Manchester involving 64 practices and 3463 patients. Tunbridge et al (1993) described an audit of 186 diabetics in four practices in Newcastle-upon-Tyne.

ML was aware of a tool (Naylor & Guyatt 1996) which can be used to appraise audit papers. Using this article we appraised the three papers (see Table 8.5).

Are the criteria valid?

The papers are published reports of multipractice audits of diabetes in primary care. Reading these papers, one thing that immediately struck us is that none of the papers reported using criteria selected following a systematic review of the literature. Criteria were developed by working parties and appeared to be based on, or extrapolated from, guidelines on the management of diabetes. We noticed that all articles consistently used certain process measures such as blood pressure recording, glycated haemoglobin measurements, and recording of smoking status, but there appeared to be some important differences. For example, the audits reported by Dunn & Bough (1996) and Tunbridge (1993) included measurement of serum creatinine, whereas Benett et al (1994) did not. We also noted that for many criteria there was insufficient information about the

Table 8.5 Critical appraisal of published diabetes audits

Criteria (Naylor & Guyatt 1996)	Dunn & Bough 1996	Tunbridge et al 1993	Benett et al 1994
Are the criteria valid?			
Was an explicit and sensible process used to identify, select and combine evidence for the criteria?	Consensus working party, based on guidelines	Consensus, working party of GPs	Working groups, adoption of British Diabetic Association guidelines as source of criteria
What is the quality of the evidence used in framing the criteria?	Insufficient information	Not explicitly stated, probably based on existing guidelines	Not explicitly stated
If necessary, was an explicit systematic reliable process used to tap expert opinion?	Insufficient information	Working party, no formal consensus methods appeared to be used	Working party, no formal consensus methods appeared to be used
Was an explicit and sensible process used to consider the relative values of different outcomes?	No	No	No
If the quality of the evidence used in originally framing the criteria was weak, have the criteria themselves been correlated with patient outcomes?	Not directly addressed	Not directly addressed	Not explicitly addressed
Were the criteria applied appropriately?	Yes	Yes	Yes
Reliable, unbiased and robust application	Yes	Yes, including explicit check for diagnostic certainty	Yes
Impact of uncertainty associated with evidence and values on the criteria-based ratings of process of care	Not addressed	Not addressed	Not addressed
Can you use the criteria in your own practice?	Yes	Yes	Yes
Are the criteria relevant to your practice setting?	Yes	Yes	Yes
Have the criteria been field-tested for use in diverse settings including settings similar to yours?	37 practices, 3974 patients, practice details not clear	4 urban GP practices	Yes

evidence base. Therefore, for all three papers, we were unable to answer the first question posed by the users' guide article: Are the criteria valid? For the second question – Were the criteria applied appropriately? – we felt that on the whole the answer was yes. As for the third question – Can you use the criteria in your own practice setting? – we felt that the answer was yes; all the audits were carried out in primary care, in large numbers of practices in different parts of the country.

From this appraisal, we felt a little more confident about our proposed audit, as we now had examples of criteria used in published audits which we could use in our own practice. A big question mark remained, however, over whether the criteria were valid. This question of the validity of the criteria used in the three published multipractice audits continued to exercise our minds. We questioned the source of the criteria and decided to investigate this further. By looking at the references cited in the papers, we identified two further papers which appeared of relevance: one was a report by the British Diabetic Association (BDA) on recommendations for the management of diabetes in primary care (BDA 1993); the second was a paper entitled 'A proposal for continuing audit of diabetes services' (Williams & Home 1992). We obtained these papers and critically appraised them using the same appraisal tool (Naylor & Guyatt 1996).

Critical appraisal of guidelines in relation to audit criteria

The BDA report is a report of a working party setting out expected standards of care for the management of diabetes in primary care. The working party consisted of a GP, a consultant physician, a public health consultant, a dietitian and a diabetes specialist nurse. It worried us that there was only one GP and no practice nurse represented. It has a specific section on recommendations for clinical audit which was of most interest to us. The document lists the process and outcome measures that should be included in an audit. The document also states that 'primary health care teams should select which criteria they wish to audit and agree the standards of care against which to audit the quality of care provided', but no guidance was provided on how to select criteria from the list.

We were aware that there are separate critical appraisal tools for clinical guidelines (described in Chapter 7), but we were much more concerned with the audit sections of the above two documents.

Next we looked at the paper by Williams & Home 1992. This is a report of a working group of the British Diabetic Association and the Royal College of Physicians. It is not clear from the paper what the composition of the panel was, but there was at least one GP in the group. A set of process and outcome measures were suggested for inclusion in the audit. However, it became clear that many of the audit measures proposed were for use in secondary care: for example, waiting and consultation times, and missed or cancelled appointments. In addition, it recommended measurement of patient satisfaction and admission rates. This paper was also critically appraised (see Table 8.6).

In summary, our exercise of appraising audit guidelines led us to conclude that none of the guidelines used an explicit process to identify evidence or to assess its quality. However, we were struck by how consistently certain process measures were recommended by the guidelines and used in the published audits, which gave us a clearer idea of what to include in our audit.

Returning to the audit in practice

It was also clear to us that some criteria were judged to be more important than others. We came up with three groups of criteria. The first group consisted of criteria which were to be definitely included in the audit (see Table 8.7); the second group we might include, but were not of the same importance as the first group (see Table 8.8); and the third group were criteria which we did not wish to use.

Criteria to be definitely included in an audit of diabetes ('Must do')

A criterion was placed in the first group on the basis of firm research evidence and impact on outcome (Baker and Fraser 1995). For example, regular assessment of diabetes control by measurement of glycated haemoglobin (or equivalent) is important, as good control prevents complications of diabetes, although the risk of hypoglycaemia increases.

Criteria that might be included ('Should do')

The second group includes criteria for which there is some research evidence for inclusion. This does not mean that

Table 8.6 Critical appraisal of guidelines for audit of diabetes

Criteria (Naylor & Guyatt 1996)	British Diabetic Association 1993	Williams & Home 1992
Are the criteria valid?		
Was an explicit and sensible process used to identify, select and combine evidence for the criteria?	Not stated – appears to be a consensus guideline	Not stated – based on selected guidelines
What is the quality of the evidence used in framing the criteria?	Insufficient information	Insufficient information
If necessary, was an explicit systematic reliable process used to tap expert opinion?	Insufficient information	Insufficient information
Was an explicit and sensible process used to consider the relative values of different outcomes?	No	No
If the quality of the evidence used in originally framing the criteria was weak, have the criteria themselves been associated with patient outcomes?	No	No
Were the criteria applied appropriately?	Not directly addressed	Not directly addressed
Reliable, unbiased and robust application	Yes	Not applicable
Impact of uncertainty associated with evidence and values on the criteria-based ratings of process of care	Not applicable	Not applicable
Can you use the criteria in your own practice?	Not directly addressed – the document states that practices should select criteria but no guidance is given as to how	Not addressed
Are the criteria relevant to your practice setting?	Yes	Some criteria, others for secondary care
Have the criteria been field-tested for use in diverse settings including settings similar to yours?	Yes – mostly, except for certain investigations such as albumin excretion rates	Some criteria, others more relevant to secondary care

they should not be included in an audit but merely that the criteria in the first group have the highest priority and must be included in all audits, whereas practices which hope to do more elaborate audits could include the second group. In some cases there may be difficulty in deriving measurable criteria. For example, we were interested in including patient education as an audit criterion, but could not work out how performance in this area could be measured in a simple way. The same applied to 'dietary review'. We were unconvinced about the value of routine measurement of renal function by serum creatinine tests, but agreed that

Table 8.7 Criteria to be definitely included in an audit of diabetes ('Must do')

- Correct diagnosis
- Glycated haemoglobin or other measure of long-term control
- Assessment of symptoms including hypoglycaemia
- Recording of smoking status
- Retinal examination through dilated pupils
- Urine for protein
- Blood pressure
- Examination of feet

Table 8.8 Criteria that might be included in an audit of diabetes ('Should do')

- Regular weighing
- Self-monitoring blood/urine
- Serum lipids
- Referrals
- Education
- Microalbuminuria
- Dietary review
- Routine renal function

further evaluation was necessary if proteinuria was detected.

Criteria not be included

We decided not to include a criterion about recording family history, as this did not seem to be an important process measure and cannot be changed. The issue of whether to do a random glucose reading when patients present at the clinic, or doing a spot urine check for glucose also exercised us. How helpful would each of these be? We decided that they would probably not give very useful information about control. We also felt that recording outcomes such as amputations would not by itself lead to improved care for diabetic patients – a diabetic patient may have received 'perfect care', but may still develop poor outcomes such as blindness or amputations through, for example, smoking or poor compliance. Therefore we were interested in using process measures for audit as they appeared to be a more sensitive measure of quality than outcome data (Brook et al 1996).

Next steps

Having agreed our essential criteria, we then decided to convene a meeting to discuss the next steps. It occurred to us that we had not sufficiently involved our practice nurse or the receptionist who was going to be help us with the audit, so they were invited to the meeting. We decided to write a protocol for our audit using the following headings:

- Aim of the audit.
- The agreed evidence-based and prioritized criteria and standards.
- Method of data collection:
  — How are patients to be identified?
  — Which types of patients are to be included?
  — What sample is to be used?
  — How will data be collected?
  — How will data collection be verified? (interrater reliability)
- Collect data.
- Analyse data and compare with target criteria and standards.
- Agree and implement changes.
- Re-audit.

We were committed to this audit and wanted to ensure a rigorous method. We wanted to be sure that there was an objective assessment of our actual performance. For help with sample size, we consulted our local audit group, who sent us a paper which contained a useful formula for calculating the sample size (Evidence-based Care Resource Group 1994).

Conclusions

The process of critical appraisal of an audit, a published audit tool and guidelines containing advice about audit criteria has been described. This process highlights the difficulties that we encountered in finding audit criteria which are evidence-based. There are very few published audits or audit tools which are sufficiently based on evidence. However, many evidence-based audit protocols developed by national centres are now becoming available through local primary care audit groups.

   Audit features so strongly in the lives of GPs that we need to have a working knowledge of an evidence-based approach to it. GPs need to acquire confidence in appraising an audit and be able to judge its quality. Clinical audit should be conducted in a rigorous, systematic manner and follow the steps outlined in Table 8.1. The most critical aspect of any audit tool is that there should be sufficient detail to enable the reader to decide whether a systematic method was used to develop the audit criteria (transparency). Any clinical audit criterion needs to be justified on the basis of research evidence. Here the rules for clinical evidence can be used to prioritize audit criteria; evidence from meta-analysis or randomized controlled trials would be accorded a higher priority than evidence from uncontrolled studies. Consensus and expert opinion are less appropriate as guides to audit but in the absence of best available evidence may be the only alternative. In addition, the setting should be taken into account; criteria for management of diabetes in secondary care may well be different from what is applicable in primary care.

References

Baker R, Fraser R C 1995 Development of review criteria: linking guidelines and assessment of quality. British Medical Journal 311: 370–373

Baker R, Hearnshaw H, Cooper A, Cheater F, Robertson N 1995 Assessing the work of medical audit advisory groups in promoting audit in general practice. Quality in Health Care 4: 234–239

Benett I J, Lambert C, Hinds G, Kirton C 1994 Emerging standards for diabetes care from a city wide primary care audit. Journal of Diabetic Medicine 11: 489–492

Bhopal R S, Thomson R 1991 A form to help learn and teach about assessing medical audit papers. British Medical Journal 303: 1520–1522

British Diabetic Association 1993 Recommendations for the management of diabetes in primary care. British Diabetic Association, London

Brook R H, McGlynn E A, Cleary P D 1996 Measuring the quality of care. New England Journal of Medicine 335: 966–970

Dunn N, Bough P 1996 Standards of care of diabetic patients in a typical English community. British Journal of General Practice 46: 401–405

Evidence-based Care Resource Group 1994 3 Measuring performance: How are we managing this problem? Canadian Medical Association Journal 150: 1575–1579

Fraser R C, Baker R, Lakhani M 1998 Evidence-based audit. Butterworth-Heinemann, Oxford (in preparation)

General Medical Council 1995 Duties of a doctor. General Medical Council London

Institute of Medicine 1992 Guidelines for clinical practice: from development to use. National Academy Press, Washington DC

Joint Audit Review Group 1995 Development of audit review tool. Eli Lilly National Clinical Audit Centre, University of Leicester

Naylor C D, Guyatt G H 1996 Users' guide to the medical literature IX. How to use an article about a clinical utilization review. Journal of the American Medical Association 275: 1435–1439

Tunbridge F K, Millar J P, Schofield P J, Spencer J A, Young G, Home P D 1993 Diabetes care in general practice: an approach to audit of process and outcome. British Journal of General Practice 43: 291–295

Williams D R R, Home P D and members of a working group of the research unit of the Royal College of Physicians and British Diabetic Association 1992 A proposal for continuing audit of diabetic services. Diabetic Education 9: 759–764

CHAPTER 9

Do antibiotics help children with otitis media?
How to use an overview

Jonathan Deeks

The clinical problem

Dr P was running a surgery in a suburban practice on the outskirts of a major city. A mother brought in her son, aged 3, with a classical presentation of acute otitis media (AOM). On examination the left tympanic membrane was red. The pain associated with the infection was making the child distressed. Whilst past experience has suggested that acute otitis media can resolve without antimicrobial treatment, Dr P was unsure whether uncomplicated AOM (a) does require treatment with antibiotics, (b) whether the symptoms would resolve quicker with a course of antibiotics, or (c) whether any benefits of giving antibiotics were outweighed by their side-effects. Dr P decided to treat the patient. She was interested in learning about how to understand and apply results from overviews. She decided to discuss her patient with JD, who has a special interest in the subject.

Formulating and contextualizing the problem

The characteristics of the patient's problem help to point the way towards an appropriate study. Sackett et al (1997) suggested that a treatment decision should be thought of in four components: the patient's problem, the suggested intervention, the alternative intervention and the desired outcomes of treatment. When looking at a question of treatment, the least biased results would be obtained from randomized controlled trials. The trials would include children with presenting symptoms similar to Dr P's patients, and would compare the suggested outcomes between two groups, one of which would have received the proposed intervention, the other an alternative intervention:

- Patient problem: child with acute otitis media

- Intervention/treatment: short course of antibiotics
- Alternative treatment: no treatment
- Desired outcomes:
  — short-term: resolution of pain and other troublesome symptoms, decrease in complications, such as perforation, acceptable side-effects of treatment
  — long-term: reduction in complications, such as conductive deafness and glue ear.

Searching for a suitable study

Dr P considered the problem and visited the local hospital library to try to find an article to help answer this query. However, a little searching revealed a plethora of relevant clinical trials. She thought it could be better to base the decision on all available evidence, rather than picking a single trial, but the prospect of critically appraising all the evidence was daunting and could not be accomplished in the short time she had to spare.

An alternative was to look for a systematic review where somebody else has done all of the work. This would give the benefits of looking at all of the appropriate data from a lot of trials without necessarily having to locate, critically appraise or understand their individual results.

An introduction to overviews

The review article has been a regular feature of medical journals for many years. Traditionally such articles have been written by experts and have described the epidemiology, diagnosis, treatment and likely outcomes of specific diseases and conditions. In the 1980s, Mulrow (1987) declared that whilst such review articles were often educational, they were commonly incomplete, opinionated and selective in the data that they referenced. For these reasons, they do not provide a sound basis for treatment decisions. Since then the systematic review has gradually emerged as an identifiable entity, aiming to produce a comprehensive overview of the results of all currently available studies, and paying special attention to the value of the data from each one. The identifiable characteristics of a systematic review are given in Table 9.1.

Systematic reviews are not limited to assessing the effectiveness of treatments. For example, systematic reviews have been used in evaluating the accuracy of diagnostic

Table 9.1 Characteristics of systematic review

- Rigourous:
  — Scientific rigour of individual studies is appraised.
  — Individual studies only included if they are unlikely to be biased.
  — Potential biases in the methods used in compiling the review assessed.
- Informative:
  — Focuses on providing an answer to a specific decision problem.
  — Presents a clear overall result with a measure of certainty.
- Comprehensive:
  — Aims to include all relevant studies
- Explicit:
  — Clearly states eligibility criteria for study inclusion.
  — Describes the methods used to locate, appraise and synthesize studies.

tests, and in assessing potential harmful effects of drugs. However, this chapter focuses on providing a framework for identifying, evaluating and interpreting the results of a systematic review of a treatment. Through the use of a specific example I will illustrate how this framework can be used to evaluate a systematic review for use in a patient's problem in general practice.

Locating systematic reviews

When looking for other papers, we usually first search the MEDLINE database to locate potentially useful articles. Dr P could follow the same route here, by producing a search strategy to look with the Medical Subject Headings (MeSH terms) 'Otitis media' and 'antimicrobials', and then limiting the search to articles with publication type 'review'. This list, however, will include all review articles, whether or not they were systematic, and locating a suitable article may take some time. Many of the unsuitable articles will be removed if the MeSH term 'meta-analysis' is added to the search. However, this will throw away some of the good stuff as well. (Meta-analysis is sometimes used as a synonym for systematic review, but properly refers to the statistical method used to combine data which is only used in a subset of systematic reviews.) Most importantly, MEDLINE does not cite any systematic reviews produced by the Cochrane Collaboration, so a MEDLINE search may not locate the most useful articles. This may change soon.

The COCHRANE LIBRARY

A preferable set of databases to search is that known as the

COCHRANE LIBRARY. These are available on a single CD-ROM and can be found in many hospital libraries in England and Wales. (If you do not have easy access, it is an inexpensive and valuable subscription for a practice library; contact details are: Update Software, P O Box 696, Oxford OX2 7YX, UK; e-mail: update@cochrane.co.uk; Web site: http://www.cochrane.co.uk.) The COCHRANE LIBRARY contains two databases that are of potential use – the COCHRANE DATABASE OF SYSTEMATIC REVIEWS (CDSR), and the DATABASE OF ABSTRACTS OF REVIEWS OF EFFECTIVENESS (DARE).

CDSR — COCHRANE DATABASE OF SYSTEMATIC REVIEWS

The CDSR contains full-text systematic reviews which have been produced by members of the Cochrane Collaboration. These reviews are only published in electronic form, which allows them to be updated regularly as new trials are located or published. All Cochrane reviews are performed according to a standard methodology, and are organized through editorial groups within the collaboration. They are also presented in a standard format by software which comes as part of the COCHRANE LIBRARY.

DARE — DATABASE OF ABSTRACTS OF REVIEWS OF EFFECTIVENESS

DARE contains abstracts of systematic review articles which have been published in medical journals. Before articles are entered on DARE they are filtered to remove review articles which do not fulfil minimal standards for systematic review. A proportion of the articles include independently written structured abstracts. The abstract contains information which will allow you to judge whether it is likely to be relevant to your question, and whether its methods are rigorous enough. However, unlike CDSR, you will need to refer to the printed journal to obtain a copy of the paper.

Searching the COCHRANE LIBRARY

To search for articles on the COCHRANE LIBRARY you click the 'search' button on the title screen. Two approaches are then possible. The first is a simple search on one term (such as 'otitis media'); the second involves choosing the

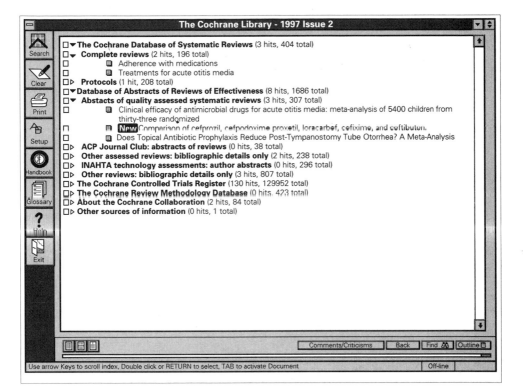

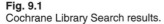

Fig. 9.1
Cochrane Library Search results.

'advanced search' option and entering a search strategy, as
would be done in MEDLINE. This would allow a search for
articles related to 'otitis media' to be restricted to those
which mention 'antibiotic'. The search engine on the
COCHRANE LIBRARY searches all the databases
simultaneously. Using an advanced search combining 'otitis
media' with 'ANTIBI*' (*is a wild card which will retrieve
all words starting with the preceding letters), we located
three articles within CDSR, and eight within DARE (see
Fig. 9.1). Two titles appear very appropriate: a Cochrane
review, subsequently published in the *British Medical Journal*
(Glasziou et al 1997, Del Mar et al 1997) and a paper
reporting a meta-analysis of randomized trials (Rosenfeld
et al 1994).

Does the review answer the question posed?

Before investing too much time in appraising and comprehending the results of the review articles, it is important to ensure that they will provide an answer to the patient problem under consideration, as we have outlined in Table 9.1. Some systematic reviews state an objective which may provide this information. However, it is better to look for a list of eligibility criteria used to determine the inclusion of studies in the review. All systematic reviews should clearly state these criteria, which often closely follow the same format as the four-part question.

Cochrane review (Glasziou et al 1997, Del Mar et al 1997)

In Cochrane reviews the eligibility criteria are stated in the 'Materials and methods' section. Four separate criteria are given: type of study, type of participant, type of intervention and type of outcome measure. Glasziou et al (1997) choose only to include randomized controlled trials (which is the case for most reviews within CDSR) which studied children suffering from AOM. The review aims to look at antimicrobial and/or surgical procedures compared to placebos. For trials to be included they had to assess success of treatment in terms of patient-orientated outcomes: in this case duration of pain, deafness, adverse effects and recurrent attacks.

Journal article (Rosenfeld et al 1994)

Rosenfeld et al (1994) also include a clear definition of eligibility criteria. They also use randomized controlled trials, and give inclusion criteria for the participants and interventions in greater detail. They do not specify what outcomes had to be presented for a study to be eligible in the same section, but later in the paper they describe two outcomes that they consider. Primary control is defined as the absence of all presenting symptoms and improvement in the appearance of the tympanic membrane (with or without a resolution of middle ear effusion and a bacteriological cure) at day 7 or day 14. Secondary control is defined as the absence of middle ear effusion 30 days after treatment.

Rosenfeld et al also include articles that make comparisons between different antibiotics.

The two reviews look as if they will both provide data that will be useful in answering our patient problem. Whilst the combined primary control endpoint in Rosenfeld et al's review initially appears a good idea, it may prove difficult to identify studies which assess such a global outcome in a standard way, so that many of the otherwise eligible randomized controlled trials may be excluded.

Are the results of the review trustworthy?

Once it has been agreed that the located publications may potentially provide an answer to the patient problem, it is necessary to appraise their validity and the degree of veracity that can be attributed to their results. Below are four criteria which should detect the major methodological shortcomings in a systematic review. At present we do not possess evidence of their relative importance, so it is not possible to judge the degree of bias avoided by each:

- Are the methods of finding, appraising and synthesizing the studies explicit?
- Is the search comprehensive?
- Was the validity of the original studies appraised and found to be adequate?
- Are the methods of assessing the literature rigorous?

Criteria

Are the methods of finding, appraising and synthesizing the studies explicit?

Good scientific articles explicitly state their methods. Review articles should state methods of literature retrieval, criteria for assessing eligibility, criteria for assessing the validity of primary studies, and the methods for pooling the individual study results. If they do not, a reader cannot judge whether or not the results of the study are trustworthy.

It is unfortunate that the tradition in review articles has been to omit all mention of methods. It seems likely that some of the review articles published without methods have been undertaken in a rigorous and scientific manner, but it is impossible to confirm or refute this.

Is the search comprehensive?

It is important that a systematic review appraises as much relevant literature as possible, and that the manner in which the search is undertaken does not introduce bias. A good review should state the literature sources and search strategies used, so that a reader can judge whether it is possible that important and potentially influential studies may have been missed.

The precision of the results depends on the number of studies included and their size. The comprehensiveness of a search can be extended by searching several electronic databases (such as MEDLINE, and other alternatives like EMBASE, which indexes more non-English language journals) using advanced searching strategies, and by making use of specialized databases (such as the COCHRANE CONTROLLED TRIALS REGISTER). Manual searching of the references of retrieved articles and bibliographies of texts may yield additional studies, as may contacting experts and researchers in the fields, and hand-searching relevant key journals.

If the ability to find articles in a search is linked to their results, then the search will be biased. A comprehensive literature search is less likely to be seriously biased than searches based around personal collections of papers, specific journals and languages. However, it is possible that some studies will be missed if they remain unpublished or have never been written up. Such publication bias is rarely as serious as it is feared to be. Research has shown that the randomized controlled trials least likely to be written up are small and have non-significant results, and hence would only contribute a small amount of information if they were being combined with larger studies. However, if a review is only combining very few studies, or studies of small to moderate size, publication bias may be a problem.

Even when comprehensive searches are undertaken, the results of a review can be irrelevant if important studies are published after the review has been written but before the review is read by people who will use its results. The use of electronic publications, such as in the COCHRANE DATABASE OF SYSTEMATIC REVIEWS, can facilitate the routine updating of reviews, so that this possibility becomes unimportant.

Was the validity of the original studies appraised and found to be adequate?

The conclusions drawn from a systematic review must reflect the strength of evidence of the original studies that it contains. Hence it is important that the quality of the individual studies is assessed. Clinical trials that are improperly randomized or where allocation schedules are not concealed from the investigators are known to give biased results. In addition, the proportion of participants who drop out of a trial, and the way in which they are accounted for in the analysis can introduce bias, as can the manner in which the outcomes are assessed. Chapter 6 of this book gives more details of these criteria.

A systematic review should assess and report on such criteria individually for each study, so that a reader can judge the degree to which the results of the primary studies could be biased. In addition, a review should state some minimal criteria which studies should meet to be included. Commonly, these detail appropriate methods of randomization, outcome assessment and acceptable dropout rates.

Are the methods of assessing the literature rigorous?

Reviewers often have to use subjective judgments when selecting relevant articles, assessing methodological quality, and extracting data. Variations in expression in research reports often lead to ambiguity, and the omission of crucial pieces of information mean that many of these decisions are not clear-cut. A good review will attempt to assess the reliability of the reviewers' decision-making process, and to investigate whether or not it could make an impact on the conclusions of the review.

Reliability can be assessed by comparing the judgments of at least two reviewers who are independently making the same decisions. The Kappa coefficient is often used to describe the degree of concordance: perfect concordance would produce a Kappa coefficient of 1; Kappas of above 0.6 are usually interpreted as indicating good agreement.

Disagreements between reviewers often arise through errors or oversights of detail, which can be quickly resolved. However, occasionally they indicate that the inclusion of an article is open to debate. A simple sensitivity analysis, where the analysis is repeated with and without these studies, can assess whether the uncertainty over inclusion could make a difference to the conclusions.

Results of validity checks

Both reviews give very detailed methods sections demonstrating that great attention has been paid to validity in their execution. However, they both searched only one database (MEDLINE), so it is possible that studies published in journals only indexed in other databases may have been omitted. Both reviews appraised the methodological quality of the studies. The Cochrane reviewers (Glasziou et al 1997, Del Mar et al 1997) tabulated the quality criteria for each study, revealing that the majority of included studies were double blind and had used an adequate method of randomization. Less than half of those included in Rosenfeld's review were double blind, and around half stated the method of randomization. Both reviews used multiple assessors to check study selection and data abstraction, but neither report on the reliability of the decision processes. In addition, both removed some identifying details from the articles in an attempt to ensure that selection was not biased by knowledge of authors, institutions or journals. More importantly, Glasziou et al removed the results sections from the papers so that selection could not be biased by knowledge of the findings.

The principles of combining data

Reviews often state that the results of the individual studies are combined using statistical methods such as Mantel-Haenszel, fixed effect, random effects, likelihood methods etc. (Deeks et al 1996). The individual details of each of these methods are not of importance to a user of reviews, but there are benefits in having an understanding of some of the basic principles by which they work.

Using summary statistics

A common misunderstanding of meta-analysis is that all the data from the individual trials are added up, and an overall effect calculated from the totals. Such an approach can yield misleading results, giving both an erroneous estimate of the treatment effect, and an overestimate of precision. In addition, such uncontrolled pooling of data from a variety of studies seems contrary to the basic premise of a good study: that of ensuring that comparisons are made between groups which are alike in all respects other than the treatment that they receive. A better approach (which all of the above methods take) is to calculate the treatment effect within each of the studies (on the basis of like-with-like comparisons), and then to average these treatment effects.

Choosing a measure of treatment effect

Most systematic reviews look at some event as being the principle outcome, and hope to see either a reduction in an event rate (if events are bad) or an increase (if they are desirable). (A rate gives the probability of someone incurring the event in the follow-up period.) The difference in event rates between the groups can be described either by dividing the rate in the treatment group by that in the control to give a relative rate (or a relative risk) or by taking the difference between the two rates (the absolute rate change). It is rare that these two alternatives lead to treatment effects in different directions. The relative rate approach is often tidier, in that relative rates are more often found to be similar in the various trials included in a systematic review than differences in absolute rates.

Another variation is to express the event rate in terms of odds rather than probabilities. This is most often done for reasons of mathematical dogma and can lead to confusion in the interpretation of results. Whilst odds ratios are known to be very similar to relative risks if events are rare, this is rarely the case in randomized controlled trials, as huge numbers need to be recruited to show a difference when event rates are very low. In situations where event rates are above 20% the interpretation of odds ratios as if they were relative rates tends to the overestimation of treatment effects.

Calculating a weighted average

The overall treatment effect is calculated by taking an average of the individual treatment effects. Usually studies are not regarded as all being equally important – studies which contain more participants should give more accurate reflections of the overall treatment effect than those with fewer participants, and deserve more weight in the analysis. The average effect is calculated weighting each trial according to a measure of its relative value. Average effects should always be quoted with a confidence interval which describes the precision (and hence infers the statistical significance) associated with the estimate of the effect of treatment.

Is the average a sensible summary of the data?

The play of chance means that we expect the results of studies to vary. However, the treatment may not be equally effective in all circumstances, so that the results of studies may also vary for reasons beyond chance. For example, the studies may have used different drug formulations, routes of administration and treatment schedules. The participants may have different disease presentations, or be from different age or ethnic groups, and the health care setting in which treatments are given may allow for different degrees of patient monitoring and care. It is also possible for treatment effects to vary systematically according to the study execution: for example, according to the method of outcome assessment or treatment allocation.

Between-study variation – heterogeneity

It is important to know whether the between-study variation is large enough to suggest that there may be important patient factors which affect treatment efficacy, and to describe how the variation could influence the review's conclusion. Some reviews may also explicitly investigate and estimate the effects of treatment modifiers.

Between-study variability is commonly termed heterogeneity. Its significance can be assessed by specific statistical tests. In systematic reviews with few studies it can be quite difficult for a heterogeneity test to reach significance, even when other factors are affecting treatment efficacy.

When significant heterogeneity is detected, the confidence interval associated with the overall treatment effect will overestimate precision. Alternative analyses using statistical methods called random effects models give more conservative results that many regard as being more appropriate in these circumstances.

There are several problems in investigating potential reasons for heterogeneity, systematic reviews not being the safest study design for investigating theories of treatment effect modification. As there are very few data points, it is remarkably easy to think up some theory which will fit in with the observed data: hence explanations which are determined prior to data analysis are regarded as more credible. In addition, even though treatment effects are estimated on the basis of randomized comparisons, participants were not randomized into one trial rather than the other, so the results of such 'between-trial' comparisons may be misleading. There will always be another explanation for the observed effects.

Methods of analysis used in the articles

Both review articles use a variety of statistical methods to combine summary statistics. The Cochrane software allows readers to make their own choice of summary statistic (odds ratio, relative risk or absolute risk difference) and statistical method (random or fixed effects). In this chapter I have chosen to express the results as relative risks, but a reader could easily make a different choice, and investigate whether it makes any difference to interpretation.

Rosenfeld et al (1994) also performed more than one statistical analysis. Whilst their main analysis estimated overall treatment effects as risk differences (combining them using a random effects analysis which overcomes the problems of between-trial variations), they also report a standard pooling of odds ratios demonstrating the robustness of their conclusions to choice of statistical method.

In addition to computing overall treatment effects Rosenfeld et al used more complex statistical methods to investigate whether there were significant differences between the studies according to the definitions of the primary control endpoint, presenting symptoms, and the antibiotics prescribed.

Interpretation of results of reviews

Graphical methods are commonly used to display the results of a systematic review. Forest plots (such as Fig. 9.3, p. 169) display both the results of the individual studies (each on a different line) and the overall results (usually below the individual study findings). The graphical display has the effect measured on the horizontal axis, with a vertical line indicating 'no effect'. Points to the left of the line relate to the treatment reducing event rates; those to the right relate to treatment increasing event rates. The results of each study are plotted using a point (indicating the observed treatment effect) and a horizontal bar (indicating the confidence interval associated with the treatment effect). The overall treatment effect is marked as a diamond at the bottom of the plot: the centre of the diamond indicates the overall effect, and its points indicate the limits of the confidence interval. If individual bars of the diamond lie entirely to the left or right of the vertical line, then that particular result is statistically significant.

Interpretation of effect size

The conclusions of a review can fall into one of four basic categories. If the overall result is statistically significant and large enough to be clinically important, then it can be concluded that the treatment is proven to do significant good or to do significant harm. If the confidence interval crosses the no-effect line, then the treatment has no effect. The remaining options are for the treatment effects to cross the no-effect line, but to include options of either significant benefit or harm, in which case the results are inconclusive, and will remain so until more research is undertaken.

Judging the clinical importance of a result expressed as a relative risk or odds ratio can be difficult. Absolute differences in rates are easier to interpret, as they can be thought of as the proportion of people that will benefit out of all those treated. Alternatively, the inverse of the absolute difference in rates gives the number of people needed to be treated for one additional person to benefit (the NNT). The formula for this was shown in Chapter 6. The same figures can be calculated from odds ratios and relative risks, if the patient's expected event rate without treatment (PEER) is known (see Table 9.2). This can often be estimated from the event rates in the control groups.

Interpretation of heterogeneity and assessment of applicability

The presence of significant heterogeneity indicates that the effect of treatment is not a simple mechanism and varies between the studies. If a random effects analysis is used, the magnitude of this variation is included in the confidence interval, which can then be interpreted as before. Even so, the lack of consistency in treatment effects may lead a reader to attribute a slightly lower strength of evidence to the results than would otherwise be the case.

The possibility of obtaining a set of heterogeneous study results in a systematic review may suggest that reviews should only be performed using very restrictive criteria, such as by a single named drug, or for patients presenting with a tightly defined group of symptoms. However, the applicability of the results of a review to a particular

Table 9.2 Conversion of odds ratios and relative risks into numbers needed to treat

1. **Converting an odds ratio (OR) into a number needed to treat (NNT)**

   a. *For decreases in event rates (OR < 1)*

   $$NNT = \frac{1 [PEER \times (1 - OR)]}{(1 - PEER) \times PEER \times (1 - OR)}$$

   b. *For increases in event rates (OR > 1)*

   $$NNT = \frac{1 + [PEER \times (OR - 1)]}{(1 - PEER) \times PEER \times (OR - 1)}$$

2. **Converting a relative risk into a number needed to treat**

   a. *For decreases in event rates (RR < 1)*

   $$NNT = \frac{1}{(1 - RR) \times PEER}$$

   b. *For increases in event rates (RR > 1)*

   $$NNT = \frac{1}{(RR - 1) \times PEER}$$

---

situation depends on inclusion of studies with similar participants in the analysis and such a derivative overview will have very limited relevance. A common strategy in systematic reviewing is to use broad inclusion criteria, as the applicability of a treatment may be established to a larger group of people if a clear benefit of treatment is noted, regardless of the presence or absence of heterogeneity.

What do the results of the two articles say?

Rosenfeld study

Rosenfeld (1994) reports two distinct sets of results. The comparisons of antibiotics with placebo treatment from four trials showed an average absolute increase of 13.1% (95% confidence interval 2.1%–24.1%) for the outcome of primary symptom control. Whilst the average increases varied between 10% and 20% for different types of antibiotics, none of the direct comparisons (from 27 additional trials) between different antibiotic types revealed significant differences. Figure 9.2 summarizes the overall findings for each of these comparisons. No placebo controlled trials report on the outcome of resolution of middle ear effusion (secondary symptom control).

The 13.1% absolute risk difference can easily be converted into a number needed to treat by taking its reciprocal, suggesting that for every 7–8 patients treated with antibiotics, one will achieve primary symptom control within 7–14 days who otherwise would not. We can get an

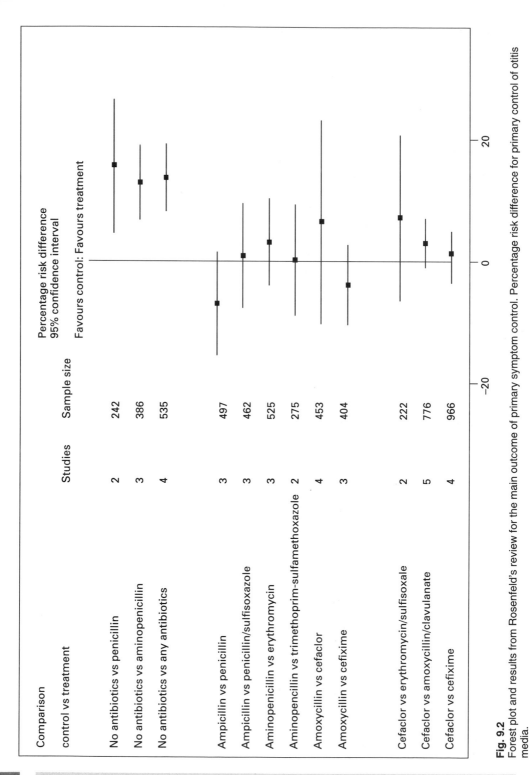

Fig. 9.2
Forest plot and results from Rosenfeld's review for the main outcome of primary symptom control. Percentage risk difference for primary control of otitis media.

idea of the recovery rate without treatment by looking at the primary control rates in the placebo groups. Rosenfeld reports this to be around 70%, but also gives a figure of 81% on the basis of a more complex statistical model. Regardless of which is correct, it appears that the majority of subjects would have recovered without treatment.

Cochrane review

Glasziou et al (1997) and Del Mar et al (1997) found eight trials comparing placebo with antibiotic treatment, which included the four placebo controlled trials pooled by Rosenfeld. The additional four trials had all been located by Rosenfeld but not included as they did not provide usable data for his definition of primary control. In fact, Glasziou failed to extract any usable data from one of them as well. Three of the trials gave data on reported pain at 24 hours, whilst six detailed reported pain at 2–7 days. Glasziou's analysis (see Fig. 9.3) revealed little effect on pain at 24 hours, but a significant reduction with antibiotics at 2–7 days (relative risk = 0.64, 95% confidence interval (0.50, 0.82)). This figure can be converted into a number needed to

Review: Treatments for acute otitis media
Comparison: Antibiotic versus placebo
Outcome: Pain

Study	Expt n/N	Ctrl n/N	Relative risk (95% fixed)	Weight (%)	RR (95% CI fixed)
Pain at 24 hours					
Burke91	53/112	56/117		43.9	0.99 [0.75, 1.30]
Thalin85	58/159	58/158		46.6	0.99 [0.74, 1.33]
vanBuchem81	13/47	11/40		9.5	1.01 [0.51, 1.99]
Subtotal (95% CI)	124/318	125/315		100.0	0.99 [0.82, 1.20]
Chi-square 0.00 (df = 2) Z = 0.08					
Pain at 2–7 days					
Burke91	20/111	29/114		21.7	0.71 [0.43, 1.18]
Halsted68	17/62	1/27		7.4	1.06 [0.50, 2.25]
Kaleida91	19/488	38/492		28.7	0.50 [0.29, 0.86]
Mygind81	15/72	29/77		21.2	0.55 [0.32, 0.94]
Thalin85	15/158	25/158		18.9	0.60 [0.33, 1.09]
vanBuchem81	4/38	3/46		2.1	1.61 [0.38, 6.77]
Subtotal (95% CI)	90/929	131/914		100.0	0.64 [0.50, 0.82]
Chi-square 4.54 (df = 5) Z = 3.49					

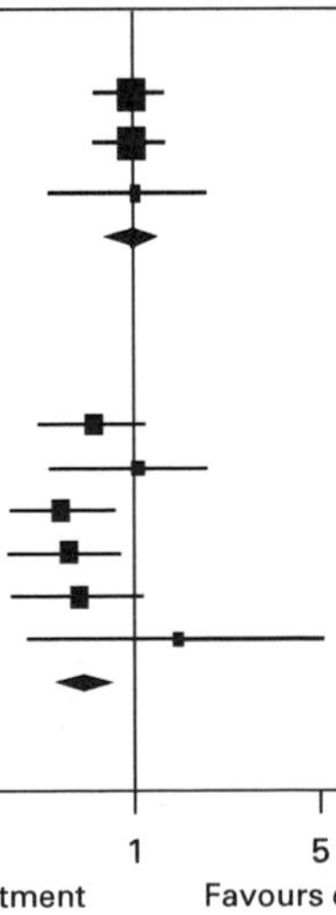

```
        0.1   0.2      1       5   10
      Favours treatment    Favours control
```

Fig. 9.3
Forest plot and results from Glasziou's review for the main outcome of resolution of pain. (df = degrees of freedom)

treat by noting that around 14% of those without treatment still had pain at 2–7 days, giving an NNT of 19.

Glasziou et al also report on five other outcomes: tympanometry, perforation, side-effects (vomiting, diarrhoea or rash), contralateral otitis and recurrences (see Fig. 9.4). Side-effects were significantly more common

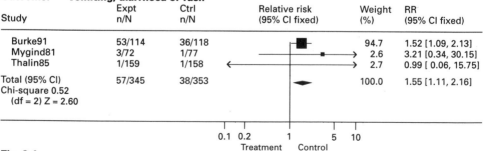

Comparison: Antibiotic versus placebo
Outcome: Tympanometry

Study	Expt n/N	Ctrl n/N	Relative risk (95% CI fixed)	Weight (%)	RR (95% CI fixed)
1 month					
Burke91	41/111	41/116		62.4	1.05 [0.74, 1.48]
Mygind81	23/72	25/77		37.6	0.98 [0.62, 1.57]
Subtotal (95% CI)	64/183	66/193		100.0	1.02 [0.77, 1.35]
Chi-square 0.04 (df = 1) Z = 0.15					
3 months					
Burke91	20/110	31/111		64.0	0.65 [0.40, 1.07]
Mygind81	18/72	18/77		36.0	1.07 [0.61, 1.89]
Subtotal (95% CI)	38/182	48/188		100.0	0.80 [0.55, 1.16]
Chi-square 1.66 (df = 1) Z = 1.17					

0.1 0.2   1   5   10
Treatment   Control

Review: Treatments for acute otitis media
Comparison: Antibiotic versus placebo
Outcome: Perforation

Study	Expt n/N	Ctrl n/N	Relative risk (95% CI fixed)	Weight (%)	RR (95% CI fixed)
Burke91	0/118	2/114		18.0	0.19 [0.01, 3.98]
Mygind81	7/72	12/77		82.0	0.62 [0.26, 1.50]
Total (95% CI)	7/190	14/191		100.0	0.55 [0.24, 1.26]
Chi-square 0.54 (df = 1) Z = 1.42					

0.1 0.2   1   5   10
Treatment   Control

Review: Treatments for acute otitis media
Comparison: Antibiotic versus placebo
Outcome: Vomiting, diarrhoea or rash

Study	Expt n/N	Ctrl n/N	Relative risk (95% CI fixed)	Weight (%)	RR (95% CI fixed)
Burke91	53/114	36/118		94.7	1.52 [1.09, 2.13]
Mygind81	3/72	1/77		2.6	3.21 [0.34, 30.15]
Thalin85	1/159	1/158		2.7	0.99 [0.06, 15.75]
Total (95% CI)	57/345	38/353		100.0	1.55 [1.11, 2.16]
Chi-square 0.52 (df = 2) Z = 2.60					

0.1 0.2   1   5   10
Treatment   Control

Fig. 9.4
Forest plots and results from Glasziou's review for secondary outcomes.

among those prescribed antibiotics (relative risk = 1.55, 95% confidence interval (1.11, 2.16), NNT = 17), whilst treatment significantly reduced rates of contralateral otitis (relative risk = 0.65, 95% confidence interval (0.45, 0.94), NNT = 13). Treatment clearly made no difference to recurrence rates. The other two outcomes showed trends towards better outcomes with treatment, but none was statistically significant. Important reductions in perforation rates with treatment could not be ruled out.

Concluding remarks

These two systematic reviews provide valuable information on the evidence concerning the use of antibiotics in acute otitis media. It is clear that a sizable proportion of cases have a quick recovery without treatment, but that treatment does speed recovery. However, a final treatment decision

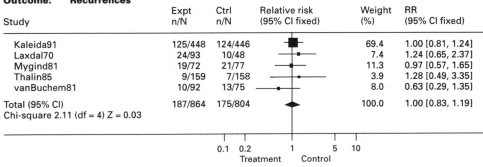

Review: Treatments for acute otitis media
Comparison: Antibiotic versus placebo
Outcome: Contralateral otitis

Study	Expt n/N	Ctrl n/N	Relative risk (95% CI fixed)	Weight (%)	RR (95% CI fixed)
Burke91	29/98	33/102		58.6	0.91 [0.60, 1.38]
Mygind81	2/72	6/77		10.5	0.36 [0.07, 1.71]
Thalin85	4/159	17/158		30.6	0.23 [0.08, 0.68]
Total (95% CI)	35/329	56/337		100.0	0.65 [0.45, 0.94]

Chi-square 6.74
(df = 2) Z = 2.31

0.1 0.2   1   5   10
Treatment   Control

Review: Treatments for acute otitis media
Comparison: Antibiotic versus placebo
Outcome: Recurrences

Study	Expt n/N	Ctrl n/N	Relative risk (95% CI fixed)	Weight (%)	RR (95% CI fixed)
Kaleida91	125/448	124/446		69.4	1.00 [0.81, 1.24]
Laxdal70	24/93	10/48		7.4	1.24 [0.65, 2.37]
Mygind81	19/72	21/77		11.3	0.97 [0.57, 1.65]
Thalin85	9/159	7/158		3.9	1.28 [0.49, 3.35]
vanBuchem81	10/92	13/75		8.0	0.63 [0.29, 1.35]
Total (95% CI)	187/864	175/804		100.0	1.00 [0.83, 1.19]

Chi-square 2.11 (df = 4) Z = 0.03

0.1 0.2   1   5   10
Treatment   Control

Fig. 9.4
Cont'd

relies on a judgement of the balance between potential benefit (control of symptoms: NNT = 8; particularly pain: NNT = 19) and possible harm (side-effects of treatment: NNT = 17). In addition there are issues regarding the prevention of worse outcomes, such as contralateral otitis or, more seriously, perforation.

The two reviews are comparable both in methods and results. However, the electronic publication approach used by the Cochrane Collaboration encourages the reporting of more outcomes than can easily be accommodated in a paper journal, which in this case reveals both the benefits and potential harms of antibiotic therapy. Electronic publication also facilitates the natural updating of systematic reviews, so that those using the information for treatment decisions will always have access to the best up-to-date evidence.

References

Deeks J J, Glanville J, Sheldon T A 1996 Undertaking systematic reviews of research on effectiveness: CRD guidelines for those carrying out or commissioning reviews. NHS Centre for Reviews and Dissemination, Report 4, University of York, York

Del Mar C, Glasziou P, Hayem M 1997 Are antibiotics indicated as initial treatment for children with acute otitis media? A meta-analysis. British Medical Journal 314: 1526–1529

Glasziou P P, Hayem M, Del Mar C B 1997 Treatments for acute otitis media in children: antibiotic versus placebo. In: Douglas R, Berman S, Black R E, Bridges-Webb C, Campbell H, Glezen P, Goodman S, Lozano J, Margolis P, Schimouchi A, Steinhoff M, Wang E, Zhu Z Acute respiratory infections module of the Cochrane Database of Systematic Reviews (updated 3 March 1997). Available in the Cochrane Library (database on disk and CD-ROM), Cochrane Collaboration, issue 2. Update Software, Oxford

Mulrow C D 1987 The medical review article: state of the science. Annals of Internal Medicine 106: 485–488

Rosenfeld R M, Vertrees J E, Carr J, Cipolle R J, Uden D L, Giebink G S, Canafax D M 1994 Clinical efficacy of antimicrobial drugs for acute otitis media: meta-analysis of 5400 children from 33 randomized trials. Journal of Pediatrics 124: 355–367

Sackett D L, Richardson W S, Rosenberg W, Haynes R B 1997 Evidence-based medicine: how to practise and teach EBM. Churchill Livingstone, New York

CHAPTER 10

Teaching and learning evidence-based practice

Peter Havelock

Introduction

The previous chapters in this book are concerned with incorporating evidence into the clinical decision-making of the primary health care team. This chapter focuses on the skills of teaching and learning evidence-based practice (EBP). The successful incorporation of evidence-based medicine (EBM) into primary care depends upon the development of the team members as both teachers and learners. It is difficult to teach on any subject without having experience in that subject. Evidence-based practice is itself a learning experience and so it is often difficult to distinguish between the roles of learner and teacher. In order to understand the importance of the relationship between the practice of evidence-based medicine and the teaching and learning of it, we first need to look into the principles behind effective learning and look into the field of education research. This chapter begins with those principles. For those who are looking for a practical guide to teaching evidence-based practice, the latter part of the chapter includes a number of ideas that have been tried and tested elsewhere.

Effective learning

A review of learning and teaching within primary care advocated a broad multifaceted approach to the teaching of evidence-based practice (Havelock et al 1995). The learning process is optimally facilitated, both practically and theoretically, by using a variety of teaching methods from a variety of sources in a variety of settings. It is essential that the learner is actively involved in making the connections across the various educational processes, thus enhancing the understanding of the information. One session on evidence-based medicine is unlikely to have any lasting effect on the behaviour of the learner.

The difficulty with the setting of general practice is that it is not generally designed for learning; it is designed for doctors to see patients and deliver health care to the population. The emphasis in many practices is on rapid performance in seeing patients rather than in learning. If we wish our trainees, GP registrars or students to learn effectively, it is important to consider how the practice can encourage rather than discourage learning. In a busy practice, learners can get the impression that 'a good GP' is always seen to be busy with patients, and that reading, thinking and learning are low priorities in a GP's life. In this context, it is difficult to persuade the trainee to learn evidence-based practice, as there is no model for learning within the practice. There is evidence of the power of modelling (Freeman et al 1982) as an important determinant of what a learner learns. If something is taught, but the learner observes contrasting behaviour by the teacher, the teacher's behaviour is most likely to be followed by the learner. The importance of modelling and the implicit, if not explicit, emphasis on performance within general practice, mean that for effective learning the teacher needs to consider what messages about learning are being transmitted by the practice.

The learning practice

If the practice is to be an effective learning environment for the trainees, GP registrars or students, it has to be an effective learning environment for all the members of the practice, and the culture of the practice needs to demonstrate this emphasis. In industry many organizations are developing themselves into 'learning organizations'. A learning organization is defined by Gavin (1993) as 'an organization that is skilled at creating, acquiring and transferring knowledge and at modifying its behaviour to reflect new knowledge'.

A learning organization is in continual development, getting value from each interaction, focusing on the team and having a clear vision of the future. It is not just about training courses, customer surveys and a glossy brochure; it is also about the culture of the organization. Garratt (1994) and Schön (1990) emphasize that the limiting factor for effective learning in many organizations is the time and emphasis given to reflection.

The ability to reflect on performance is the basis of a learning practice. It takes time and the will to develop a practice into an effective place for learning. As mentioned earlier, an emphasis on performance, without time for reflection about that performance, leads to a lost opportunity for learning and transmits the message to the learner that thinking and questioning are not part of the job. How to develop and maintain an effective learning environment will be covered in the following sections.

Structures and processes that encourage learning within the practice

In previous chapters the authors described five stages for the effective practice of EBP:

- the conversion of a problem into an answerable question
- a search for information
- critically appraising the papers
- applying the answer to the problem
- evaluating the practitioner's own performance in EBP.

I will start at the second stage and return to the conversion of a problem into a question later in the chapter.

The search for information

There is no shortage of information for a general practitioner. The amount of written material arriving unsolicited through the door has often been described in terms of feet per month or pounds per week. It is often tempting to regard this material as source of evidence. Royal College of General Practitioners examiners remember a number of candidates quoting the weekly GP broadsheets as the basis for a clinical decision. These candidates had acquired some information but had made no attempt to appraise it critically. Many practitioners regard the large amount of free magazines and journals arriving in practice as having some value. This results in little of value being read, because GPs are overwhelmed by the total amount. *Both the quality and quantity of the incoming written material make it imperative that the practitioner who is practising and teaching EBP is selective about what is read and what is kept.*

Using evidence in different ways

There are three ways of using evidence, and an effective

teaching practice needs to be able to understand and use all three methods. This flexibility of usage will save time and energy and allow the efforts made to be more effective:

1. using original articles
2. the application of evidence-based summaries
3. evidence-based practice protocols.

1. Using original articles

The use of original articles is described in a number of chapters in this book. In Chapter 2 the range of databases and the process of running an effective search are fully described. With the ease of access to the database MEDLINE from the British Medical Association library by computer and modem, the first of these criteria is comparatively easily met by most teaching practices. Most practices also have access to a local postgraduate library and the expertise and information therein.

However, using this 'prime method' of gathering information from original articles may not be straightforward. It requires the development of searching skills, access to the database, and time. It is thus at this stage that many potential evidence-based practitioners stumble and retreat into anecdote. An answer for many practitioners is the librarian in the local postgraduate medical library. The skills, willingness and availability of librarians can vary, but my experience of a wide range of postgraduate centres is that they provide a rich and willing source of untapped help and expertise. In some regions, the librarians are part of a network of health care libraries and they have put out information about how they can help the clinicians. It starts:

- You are the customer.
- You deserve a high-quality service.
- Make sure that you ask for it.

They go on to describe the help that they can give to find evidence.

Library staff can answer a wide range of inquiries at a number of levels:

- simple questions about books or reports
- literature searches combining a range of concepts
- more complex searches.

They can help you to do it yourself if you prefer, and can also obtain articles from:

- the library's own stock
- interlibrary loan
- downloading from databases.

They provide training in information-handling and searching skills.
Remember: if in doubt, ask.
With this degree of expert backup behind most general practitioners, the first stages of information-handling and searching are accessible and provide the basis for evidence-based practice.

2   The application of evidence-based summaries
Seeking and applying evidence-based summaries is a use of evidence that is open to all general practitioners. There are two information sources: the first is a new type of journal of secondary publication. Appropriate articles are selected from a wide range of journals, critically appraised, and summarized into readable form along with the appraisal. These can appeal to a general readership and many of the articles are appropriate to general practice. Examples are: the *ACP Journal* in North America and Evidence-based Medicine published by the *British Medical Journal* (now brought together in 'Best Practice' on CD-ROM), and *Bandolier*, an excellent monthly journal produced in Oxford:

> Bandolier
> Pain Relief Unit
> The Churchill
> Oxford [OX3 7LJ]
> Fax: 01865 226 1978
> Tel: 01865 226132
> e-mail:andrew.moore@pru.ox.ac.uk

These journals package information in a way that encourages readers to consider their own practice in relation to the subject matter.
   There are a number of bulletins that produce evidence-based, critically appraised summaries of a number of specific subjects that are of interest to general practitioners. These include *Effective Health Care*, published by Nuffield Institute for Health (Leeds) and the NHS Centre for Reviews and Dissemination (York):

> Effective Health Care
> NHS Centre for Reviews and Dissemination
> University of York
> York

YO1 5DD
Tel: 01904 433634
Fax 01904 433661
e-mail: neudis@york.ac.uk

Recent subjects have included: benign prostatic hyperplasia, aspirin and myocardial infarct, and the management of menorrhagia. Another journal in this range is *MeReC Bulletin*, published in Liverpool:

MeReC Bulletin
National Prescribing Centre
The Infirmary
70 Pembroke Place
Liverpool
L69 3GF
Tel: 0151 794 8130 (director)
Fax: 0151 794 8139
email: barton@liv.ac.uk(director)

In the latter are included subjects such as: hormonal contraception, non-insulin dependent diabetes, and pain control in terminal care. The fourth journal is the long-standing *Drug and Therapeutics Bulletin*, produced in London:

Drug and Therapeutics Bulletin
Consumer's Association
2 Marylebone Road
London
NW1 4DF
Tel: 0171 830 6000
Fax: 0171 830 6220
e-mail: dtb@which.net

This bulletin offers guidance to doctors in the area of therapeutics. All these publications produce well-written independent résumés of the literature available on a particular subject, including the references for the reader who wishes to take the subject further. They provide a valuable source of information for a practice that is considering its care in a particular area, or for a practitioner who wishes to keep up-to-date.

A second source of information that provides systematic reviews of a subject is the Cochrane Collaboration. This is a rapidly growing international group of clinicians and others involved in health care, who collaborate to produce systematic reviews of therapy which are frequently updated as new and relevant articles are published. The reviews are published on computer diskette or compact disc, on the Internet and in a variety of paper forms: for example, EBM journals. This is becoming an increasingly useful source of 'expert' opinion incorporating all the published work in particular areas. An example of a Cochrane review was provided in Chapter 9. More and more postgraduate libraries have access to the Cochrane database, and this is available to local general practices.

3. Evidence-based practice protocols
The third way of utilizing evidence in practice is by recourse to evidence-based protocols. These require neither the same level of skills or time as seeking original articles, nor the interpretation of evidence-based summaries into practical care. There are many protocols for care in general practice which stem from a wide number of sources. Sometimes the provider has a vested interest which becomes apparent in the protocol: for example, a pharmaceutical company wishing to increase sales of its product; a health authority wishing to reduce costs; or the local health trust wishing to influence the use of its services.

There are some national protocols that are based on evidence that come from a consensus of experts. As described in Chapters 7 and 8, local groups of GPs review the literature in certain subjects and produce locally based protocols. It is important not to reinvent the wheel, but use already recognized national guidelines in the development of local ones.

Information sources near and far

I have already discussed the central part the local postgraduate library can play in the practice of EBM, as a source of both information and skill. What place is there for a practice library in a teaching practice? Much has been written in the past about the structure and function of a practice library, but a book can become outdated even before it arrives in the bookshop. The main advantage of maintaining an up-to-date practice library is the ease of access to all members of the primary health care team at the time when the information is needed. Filed, indexed copies of the more recent issues of journals like the *BMJ*, *BJGP* and *Evidence-based Medicine* can also be helpful for immediate access to useful articles when discussing issues in the practice.

Books in a practice library play less of a part in the

practice of EBM, but have a wider role in the broader general education of trainees. Textbooks, though useful when bought, can go out of date very rapidly. Probably the most important part that the practice library plays in EBP is as an updated source of evidence-based summaries and protocols providing information for a discussion in many clinical areas. As more electronic sources of information become available to practices, and practitioners become more skilled in using them, EBM based in the practice will become more of a practical possibility.

Critical appraisal of the information

The stages and skills required to undertake critical appraisal of the information collected have been described in previous chapters. There is often a mistaken belief that critical appraisal is dependent on a detailed understanding of statistics. The main concern is, 'Are these results valid to my practice and are the conclusions applicable to my patients?' For the teacher in practice, these questions should be asked of each published guideline which sets out to encourage GPs to change their practice. Critical appraisal skills can be encouraged in our learners by all members of the practice team practising this critical approach.

Putting the ideas into practice

This is the area, both in audit and in establishing evidence-based practice, that is crucial to the whole programme. Unless behaviour changes, nothing changes. It is also the aspect that is often given the smallest amount of attention, probably because it is the most difficult task to do well. If a teacher in general practice is to encourage learners to practise EBM, it is essential that some time and effort is spent exploring what makes for effective change management.

Rogers (1983) emphasized the need to remember the three important aspects of any change when planning its implementation:

- the organization of the team
- the people involved
- the change itself.

The organization of the primary health care team

The speed of change in the National Health Service has been

rapid, and in many aspects it has been imposed on practices. This has led to many doctors and practice members feeling overwhelmed and unable to cope with more change; yet change within the health service is likely to continue to take place as rapidly, if not more rapidly. The introduction of EBP into this environment needs planning, taking into particular account the possible feelings and attitudes to change that currently exist within the practice. To help people change their clinical care, the systems within the practice need to be reviewed, the people involved need to be part of the decision-making process, and there needs to be a high level of communication between all concerned.

The people involved

Individuals react to change in different ways but there seem to be some consistent features. Whatever the change proposed, however beneficial it is, an element of loss is felt by the people involved. For example, in getting married, people lose some of their freedom; in moving into new practice premises, people lose the comfort of their old space and the security of old working conditions. The losses concerned with implementing new ideas can be related to:

- Security: people are unsure of what the future holds.
- Competence: people feel they do not have the skills to do the new job or take on the new task.
- Relationships: familiar relationships can disappear or become distant.
- Sense of direction: sometimes the direction in which people are going is not clear, and the meaning of their job might change.
- Territory: people often have a feeling of uncertainty about the area of work that used to belong to them.

Each of these losses can have costs, and people need help to cope with the grief associated with them.

There is natural resistance by most people to change; they can lose the familiar and the future becomes uncertain. This often produces patterns of behaviour which are important to recognize in both ourselves and others.

- Denial: the initial reaction is for a person to pretend the change is not happening.
- Resistance: this can be passive (just not following the required pattern of behaviour) or active (grumbling,

becoming angry, exhibiting behaviour that will block the change).
- Exploration: here people try aspects of the change, work with it, and if successful arrive at the final stage of commitment.
- Commitment: where people commit themselves to the plan and work in new ways.

Each of these stages needs recognition and active management within the practice. Individuals often do not resist change but they do resist being changed.

The change itself

Rogers (1983) described how practitioners in any field confront changes, his ideas can be applied to the introduction of the practice of evidence-based decision-making itself:

- Relative advantages: the change proposed is clearly better than the status quo.
- Compatibility: the new way of working will fit in easily with old patterns of working.
- Complexity: the changes proposed are understandable and achievable by the people who need to take them on.
- Suitability for trial: to help people accept a change, it can be taken on in stages and each stage can be evaluated.
- Observability: the process of change is clear to all those concerned with it.

There are many examples in the management and business literature (Harvey-Jones 1989, Kanter 1985) of achieving change within an organization, from which primary health care staff can learn a great deal. Key messages are:

- Involve people in the change at an early stage.
- Have a good reason to make the change.
- Put a respected person in charge of the change.
- Plan the change throughout the practice.
- Provide training if necessary.
- Install systems within the practice that maintain the change.
- Acknowledge and reward people.
- Provide clear leadership.

These messages from industry are equally applicable to general practitioners and members of the primary health care team. The lessons learnt have been applied to primary care (Spiegal et al 1992, Pringle 1993, Havelock 1995), and they would be of value to those who are wishing to bring about change within their own practices.

Practical ways of developing evidence-based learning in a practice for all team members

The most important factor in teaching evidence-based practice is for the learner to see it in action within the surgery, within the consulting room and in practice meetings. It is thus vital for the clinicians within the practice, the GPs and nurses, to be seen as learners as well as teachers, so their continuing education needs to be planned with as much care as that of the other learners, GP registrars or students. Ideally, the GP's continuing medical education or professional development would be planned as a combination of individual and practice needs. With this atmosphere within the practice – identifying and analyzing need, gathering information and planning provision based on need – evidence-based practice and learning can become the obvious way forward.

The teaching environment

Earlier in this chapter I described a model for the learning practice which is based on the literature about learning in a business organization. How can this be achieved within our own practices, organizations that are primarily designed for patient care and not for learning or teaching? For the last 2 years at the Oxford Experienced Trainers Course, I have been gathering examples of 'good practice' and 'good ideas' for developing an effective learning environment within a teaching practice; these are shown in Table 10.1.

Many of these ideas seem to have no direct relevance to teaching or practising EBM: for example, celebration of good practice, or improving patient feedback. The connection becomes more obvious, however, if EBP is related to trying to achieve 'best practice' for the patients, and so a patient focus to care provides the link. The celebration of success helps to motivate and encourage a team to work together towards 'best practice'. The achievement of an optimal learning practice needs skilled and coordinated leadership from the doctors and practice manager.

Table 10.1 The 2-year vision of the learning environment

- Improved library facilities:
  - Databases online
  - Librarian / cataloguing
  - More up-to-date books (system for purchase)
- Improved practice teamworking:
  - Common aims in management, clinical and educational
  - Mutual respect
  - Defined roles
  - Involving team expertise in teaching
  - Effective team meetings
    achieve aims
    no antagonism
    respect and building of team members
    promote enthusiasm
    produce appropriate action
    effective use of time
- Research in practice – pursuing questions and exhibiting enthusiasm:
  - Established patterns of research / published articles
  - Support, encouragement and time allowed for research
  - Research network and presenting at conferences
  - Multidisciplinary research involving the trainee
- Quality measurement and assurance:
  - Agreed standards
  - Measuring outcomes
  - Continuous and ongoing
  - Audit as a dynamic tool with all practice members
- Involving the partners in teaching:
  - Time for teaching
  - Responsibility for the trainee
  - Ongoing education for the whole practice
  - Development of the training practice ethos with support and development of the non-trainer partners
  - Development of the 'educational manager'
  - Identifying training needs within the practice as part of an ongoing plan
- Management systems:
  - Appraisal systems for all
- Improve patient feedback:
  - Focus groups of patients
  - Patient satisfaction surveys
- Celebration of good practice:
  - A congratulation book
  - Social events within the practice
- Effective leadership within the practice:
  - Partners investing in leadership / management training
  - Looking after the emotional needs involved in training the team members
  - Teaching skills training for all practice members

Evidence-based practice in the daily running of the practice

As described in Chapter 2, throughout the working day of each and every clinician there emerge problems and issues to which there is no immediately clear answer. Mostly these problems are ignored, for all the reasons that busy clinicians give for continuing to practise in the same way as they always have done. For a practice to utilize these problems as opportunities to develop their care, a number of systems can be introduced. For the problems to become useful, they need to be highlighted and changed into puzzles that then can be made into questions.

The transfer of a problem into a question

Techniques that some practices use for this process are as follows:

1. Case discussion amongst the clinicians, with the focus on the issues of care that could be improved.
2. Critical incident analysis: discussion within the practice of critical incidents, i.e. deaths, cancer diagnoses, heart attacks and strokes, and complaints, and a search for ways of improving. Both these discussion techniques can lead to many questions and a search of the literature will be needed to answer them.
3. A running notice board or flip-chart for anyone to note down a question that has come up in the course of a day's work. Examples might be:
   — Why are we doing breast checks for our patients on HRT? Is there any value in it?
   — What should be our first line of treatment for patients with mild/moderate hypertension? What lifestyle changes make any difference to blood pressure?
4. The review and questioning of current 'truths' or guidelines within the practice.
5. Practice meetings can generate a list of 'unsolved problems' or puzzles, with an action plan to find the information necessary to addressing them.

This list is by no means exhaustive and clinicians can continue to develop these ideas for encouraging curiosity and questioning within their own practice.

The place of research as a stimulus to EBP

A practice actively engaged in research is likely to use the same critical skills to review and improve patient care. Sometimes, however, the converse is true and a doctor can concentrate so much on the detail of specific research, that skills and patient care can suffer. The balance can be achieved by developing the practice into one that encourages research, particularly multidisciplinary research between doctors and nurses. This stimulates academic communication, and the information-gathering and appraisal skills that are the basis of evidence-based practice. Within this atmosphere of enquiry the learners, GP registrars and students, will gain the skills and incentive to do their own project work. In many localities multidisciplinary networks of practitioners interested in research are emerging to support research and the use of research within primary care.

EBP in the tutorial or teaching session

The tutorial or teaching session is an extension of practice learning, personalized to the individual learner, and should highlight all those messages described earlier in this chapter. Specifically, the same techniques used for the practice as a whole can be personalized for the learner. Examples might be:

- Issues raised in a tutorial can be made into questions suitable to be answered by a literature search.
- If the teaching session occurs in a place where literature is readily available, issues can be looked up at the time.
- The use of 'education prescriptions' (Evidence-based Medicine Working Group 1992), used by GP registrars in the form of their learning log (Havelock et al 1995), promote the continuation and follow-up of problems identified and solutions found.
- Project work, now a requirement for summative assessment, can be a great stimulus to developing EBP skills if used effectively.
- A skilled and prepared teacher, aware of the current literature in some of the key areas of general practice, can speed up the process of the literature search and help develop the learner's critical appraisal skills at an early stage.

It will be obvious that effective teachers of EBP should not only have the necessary knowledge and skills; they also need to be active practitioners themselves. How can a teacher develop these skills, and how should the need for these skills affect the teacher/trainer/tutor development programmes now running in the UK?

Teacher development

The first requirement of teaching EBP is to manage one's

clinical practice using evidence as the basis. In Chapter 1 both the reasons for this and many of the barriers to it are described. An awareness of these barriers is important to all potential teachers of EBP, both for themselves and their learners. The barriers to teaching EBP are similar to the barriers to practising it (EBM Working Group 1992):

1. To many learners, the skills of critical appraisal are rudimentary and EBP may thus seem threatening. Sometimes, the clinical appraisal skills of the learners are greater than those of some of the traditional teachers, with similar threats to the self-esteem of teachers!

2. People like quick and easy answers. Cookbook medicine has its appeal. The time and effort required to collect and appraise evidence may be perceived as inefficient and distracting from the real goal (to provide optimal care for patients).

3. For many clinical questions high-quality evidence is lacking. If such questions predominate when we attempt to introduce EBP, a sense of futility can result.

4. The concepts of EBP are met with scepticism by many senior doctors and teachers.

Overcoming barriers and developing teaching skills

The methods of practising and teaching EBP, as described earlier in this chapter and in previous ones, can ameliorate and reduce these barriers. If the key to teaching EBP is practising EBP, then how does a practising GP teacher develop the skills of both practice and teaching? There are a number of local and national resources which can assist. Many general practice and public health departments throughout the country have the skills of critical appraisal and will make them available to primary care team members. In Oxford, the public health department developed CASP (critical appraisal skills programme) courses for a range of health workers. These are half-day workshops to introduce participants to the key skills needed to find and make sense of evidence to support health service decisions. The workshops concentrate particularly on the critical appraisal of systematic resources and introduce people to the related ideas of the Cochrane Collaboration. CASP workshops are now spreading around the country and are a great starting point for those wishing to develop EBP skills. Further information about CASP can be obtained from:

Katie Crook or Claire Spittlehouse:
Tel: 01865 226968
Fax: 01865 226959
e-mail: Casp@eix.compulink.Co.UK
Web site: http://Fester.his.path.cam.acuk/phealth/
caspholme/htn

For those who want to develop their skills in teaching EBM
further, workshops are run by the Centre for Evidence-
based Medicine in Oxford and at University College in
London. These are week-long workshops run twice a year
for any health care worker in the NHS. The workshop is a
mixture of brief lectures, small group work, practical
teaching, searching computer databases and discussion. It is
aimed at clinicians and other health care professionals who
already have some knowledge of critical appraisal and some
experience in practising evidence-based health care, and
who want to explore issues around teaching it. Information
can be obtained from:

Programme Manager for Education and
Communication
NHS R&D Centre for Evidence-based Medicine
University of Oxford
John Radcliffe Hospital
Headington
Oxford
OX3 9DU
Tel: 01865 221321
Fax: 01865 222901
Web site: http://cabm.jrz.ox.ac.uk/docs/
workshopsteching.html

Evidence-based teachers' courses

Teaching evidence-based practice can often be seen as an
extra to teaching courses and teachers' development.
Ideally, it should be seen as the key thread running through
both practice and teaching. Our courses for GP registrars,
teachers and university tutors need to become evidence-
based. There is a wealth of information about the
effectiveness or non-effectiveness of teaching, as there is
about the effectiveness of medical interventions. This
information should be used, and should be seen to be used,
in the development of teachers, just as medical evidence is
used to develop effective doctors. Doing so would
emphasize the importance of questioning current teaching

practice, gathering and critically appraising information, and putting ideas into practical teaching. The barriers and solutions to those barriers encountered in this method of teacher development are similar to those involved in the development of evidence-based clinical practice. It is important for those of us that have responsibility for the development of teachers in primary care to practise evidence-based teaching.

Evidence-based day-release courses and continuing medical education

Many of the messages in this chapter have been targeted on teachers within general practices. They are equally relevant for course organizers, clinical tutors, GP tutors and undergraduate teachers. EBP should not be seen as one or two sessions in a programme, sandwiched between 'diabetes' and 'the consultation'. The use of information and its critical appraisal needs to be *integral* to the whole course. A learning session on 'asthma' or 'the consultation' should include searching for relevant papers on the subjects and a discussion about the validity of the evidence. There will need to be specific time available for acquiring skills in searching and critical appraisal, but these skills need to be reinforced by subsequent sessions which utilize them. Using these techniques throughout the day-release course or the refresher course will challenge the tutors. They may need to acquire specific skills on the hoof or by attending a course for teachers of evidence-based practice.

In some teaching sessions there will be prepared papers and handouts, and time for a literature search and for reading and reflection will be usual practice. Sessions will generate questions, with learners agreeing to find information for the group. Subsequent sessions will include a review of the questions from previous weeks, and the information which has been gathered will be appraised and discussed. This has implications for the professional development of course organizers and GP tutors. They need help to develop the skills of EBP and need to have experience within their own teaching of how to use these skills.

The special needs of students

Many medical schools are incorporating the teaching of evidence-based learning into their curriculum. It is also important that primary care departments and the teachers within the community adopt these methods. It was stated in Chapter 1 that many aspects of primary care lack evidence of effectiveness. There is, none the less, a considerable body of research that is applicable to daily practice, and medical students need to be made aware of this. If students are not, they may well conclude that this part of their medical course is intellectually unchallenging and thin. The development of the skills of the community teachers attached to each department needs to be provided for, so there will be some consistency in the messages given to students, whether they are out in the practices, in the lecture theatre, or in a tutorial room.

Conclusions

- It is difficult to teach EBP without practical experience of evidence-based practice.
- Educational research evidence can be useful in indicating effective teaching/learning methods.
- Learners model themselves on their teachers.
- Developing a practice that is evidence-based is, therefore, essential for an effective teacher of EBP.
- Information sources are multiple and varied, and accessible to most general practitioners. The local postgraduate library is generally a rich source of help.
- Putting new ideas into practice is difficult, and needs to be planned using evidence from primary care and from industry and management sciences.
- There are many ways of developing evidence-based learning, and they need to be integrated into everyday practice and teaching.
- Teachers in general practice, trainers, undergraduate tutors, course organizers and GP tutors need professional development in the field of EBP and in teaching EBP.

References

Evidence-based Medicine Working Group 1992 EBM: A new approach to teaching the practice of medicine. Journal of the American Medical Association 268: 2420–2425

Freeman J, Roberts J, Medcalf D, Hillier V 1982 The influence of trainers on trainees in general practice. General Practice Occasional paper, Royal College of General Practitioners, London

Garratt B 1994 The learning organisation. Harper Collins, London

Gavin D 1993 The learning organisation. Harvard Business Review 71: 78–91

Harvey-Jones J 1989 Making it happen – reflections on leadership. Fontana/Collins, London

Havelock P B 1995 Communication skills and teamworking in primary care. Publishing Initiatives, Beckenham

Havelock P, Hasler J, Flew R, McIntyre D 1995 Professional education for general practice. Oxford University Press, Oxford

Kanter R 1985 The change masters – corporate entrepreneurs at work. Unwin, London

Pringle M (ed.) 1993 Change and teamwork in primary care. British Medical Journal Publishing, London

Rogers E M 1983 Diffusion of innovations. Free Press, New York

Schön D A 1990 Educating the reflective practitioner. Josey-Bass, San Francisco

Spiegal N, Murphy E, Kinmouth A L, Ross F, Bain J, Coates R 1992 Managing change in general practice: a step-by-step guide. British Medical Journal 304: 231–234

Glossary

Terms used in therapeutics

We will discuss 2 examples to define the terms we use to denote the efficacy of treatments (1). First, for intensive therapy for diabetes mellitus (DM), the experimental event rate (EER) for neuropathy was 3% compared with the control event rate (CER) of 10% (2). Second, the home delivery of thrombolysis for myocardial infarction (MI) led to 83% survival at 30 months compared with 68% survival for delivery after transfer to hospital (3). We can then generate the measures below.

1. When the experimental treatment reduces the risk for a bad event

RRR (relative risk reduction): the proportional reduction in rates of bad events between experimental and control participants in a trial, calculated as |EER – CER| / CER. and accompanied by a 95% confidence interval (CI). In the DM example, |EER – CER| / CER = |3% – 10%| / 10% = 70%, CI 34% to 87%.

ARR (absolute risk reduction): the absolute arithmetic difference in event rates, |EER – CER|. In the DM example, |EER – CER| = |3% – 10%| = 7%.

NNT (number needed to treat): the number of patients who need to be treated to achieve one additional favourable outcome. Reported as a whole number, calculated as 1/ARR, rounded up to the next highest whole number, and accompanied by its 95% CI. In the DM example, for neuropathy, 1/ARR = 1/7% = 14.3, rounded up to 15, 95% CI 9 to 35. Readers can convert this to an NNT for a specific patient by estimating that patient's

susceptibility (patient expected event rate, or PEER, also called the patient-specific baseline risk) relative to the average control patient in the trial report, expressed as a decimal fraction (F) and then dividing the reported NNT by F. In the example, if a patient was judged to be half as susceptible as the average control patient, F = 0.5 and NNT/F = 15/0.5 = 30, then 30 such patients would need to be treated to prevent 1 additional event.

2. When the experimental treatment increases the probability of a good event

RBI (relative benefit increase): the increase in the rates of good events, comparing experimental and control patients in a trial, also calculated as |EER – CER| / CER. In the MI example, |EER – CER| / CER = |83% – 68%| / 68% = 22%.

ABI (absolute benefit increase): the absolute arithmetic difference in event rates, |EER – CER|. In the MI example, |EER – CER| = |83%–68%| = 15%.

NNT: this is calculated as above, 1/15% = 7, and denotes the number of people who must receive the experimental treatment to create one additional improved outcome in comparison with the control treatment.

3. When the experimental treatment increases the probability of a bad event

RRI (relative risk increase): the increase in rates of bad events, comparing experimental patients to control patients in a trial, and

Continued →

Glossary

calculated as for RBI. RRI is also used in assessing the impact of risk factors for disease.

ARI (absolute risk increase): the absolute difference in rates of bad events, when the experimental treatment harms more patients than the control treatment. ARI is also used in assessing the effect of risk factors for disease.

NNH (number needed to harm): the number of patients who, if they received the experimental treatment, would lead to 1 additional person being harmed compared with patients who receive the control treatment, and calculated as 1/ARI.

Confidence intervals

The confidence interval (CI) quantifies uncertainty (4). The 95% CI is the range of values within which we can be 95% sure that the true value lies for the whole population of patients from whom the study patients were selected. The CI narrows as the number of patients on which it is based increases. We prefer CIs to *P* values because the former tell us about the strength of evidence, whereas the latter merely test it against a no difference (null) hypothesis.

Odds ratio

When used to summarise a systematic review or an individual study of treatment, an odds ratio (OR) describes the odds of a patient in an experimental group having an outcome event relative to a patient in a control group (5). For example, 100 patients (a + b) receive an experimental treatment and 20 of them (a) experience an event, while 80 do not (b), whereas 100 patients (c + d) receive a control treatment and 40 have an event (c), while 60 do not (d). The odds in the experimental group is (a/b =) 0.25, the odds in the control group is (c/d =) 0.67, and the odds ratio is [(a/b)/(c/d) = 0.25/0.67)] = 0.37. Note that the odds ratio looks like a relative risk, but it is numerically similar only when event rates are very low. Thus, the relative risk for the example is [a/(a + b) + c/(c + d) = 20/100 + (40/100 =)] 0.50. If the event rates were 1% and 2%, the RR would still be 0.5, and the OR would be (1/99 + (2/98 =) 0.49. The OR is also used in other comparative studies, for example, of diagnosis, prognosis, or etiology.

References

1. Sackett D L 1996 Evidence-Based Medicine. Jan-Feb; 1: 37–8
2. Intensive glycaemic control prevented or delayed diabetic neuropathy [Abstract]. 1995 Evidence-Based Medicine. Nov-Dec; 1: 9
3. Prehospital thrombolytic therapy reduced mortality in acute MI [Abstract]. ACP J Club. 1996 Jul-Aug; 125: 6. Evidence-Based Medicine Jul–Aug; 1: 138
4. Altman D G 1996 Evidence-Based Medicine. May–Jun; 1: 102–4.
5. Sackett D L, Deeks J J, Altman D G 1996 Evidence Based Medicine. Sep–Oct; 1: 64

From: Evidence-Based Medicine Jan. Feb 1998 Vol 3, No 1, pp. 1–32.

Index